STRUCTURE OF THE HUMAN BRAIN

STRUCTURE OF THE HUMAN BRAIN A Photographic Atlas

STEPHEN J. DeARMOND, Ph.D.
The Medical College of Pennsylvania
Philadelphia, Pennsylvania

MADELINE M. FUSCO, Ph.D.
Professor
Department of Anatomical Sciences
State University of New York at Stony Brook

MAYNARD M. DEWEY, Ph.D.
Professor and Chairman
Department of Anatomical Sciences
State University of New York at Stony Brook

NEW YORK   OXFORD UNIVERSITY PRESS   LONDON   TORONTO   1974

CONTENTS

ACKNOWLEDGMENTS

We are grateful to the many students and colleagues at the Medical College of Pennsylvania (MCP) and the State University of New York Medical School at Stony Brook (SUNY) for their help and encouragement in preparing this book. We especially wish to remember with warmth and gratitude the late Miss Vera Menough who directed the histology laboratory in the Anatomy Department at MCP for over 30 years. She prepared the high quality transverse sections of the spinal cord and brain stem without which the atlas could not have been begun and taught us to prepare sections of equal quality so that the atlas could be expanded and completed. We thank Dr. David Dunn and Dr. Theordore Krouse of the Pathology Department at MCP for providing the many brain specimens needed to prepare the coronal and sagittal sections. Dr. Rosalie Burns of the Neurology Department at MCP generously provided the radioangiograms. We are grateful to Dr. Andrew Beasley for his continuing support by providing the facilities and materials to complete the majority of the work in the Anatomy Department at MCP. We would also like to thank Mr. George Boykin and Mr. David Colflesh at SUNY. Mr. Boykin provided us with the excellent specimens of the gross brain, which appear in the first section of the atlas, and Mr. Colflesh provided the fine photographs of those specimen. We especially appreciate the help of Dr. Ronald Irving who prepared the dissected specimens of the brain stem that appear in this atlas and, more importantly, critically reviewed the atlas through extensive classroom usage at both MCP and SUNY.

Finally, we are grateful to William Halpin of Oxford University Press for his sustained interest and enthusiasm for the work during the long and arduous years spent in making this atlas and to Jeffrey House for seeing the project to its completion with a strong commitment to quality.

INTRODUCTION

This atlas originally developed out of the need to provide some means by which medical students could acquire a knowledge of the structure and organization of the human nervous system in an intensified curriculum that substantially reduced the time allocated to the study of neuroanatomy in the laboratory. Thus we devised a photographic atlas consisting of large, clear, detailed reproductions of histological sections of the spinal cord and brain stem. Each photomicrograph was accompanied by a labeled diagram of the section on a facing page. This was then used by the students as a self-study visual aid, and we facilitated its use as such by means of projected slides of the photographs in lectures and demonstrations. The students liked this approach, and we found that it helped us convey to them an appreciation of the structure and organization of the human brain.

Encouraged by this experience, we have expanded the original atlas to its present form. It now provides several different views of the gross brain and of transverse, coronal, horizontal, and sagittal planes of section of the neuroaxis. Most of the sections are paired: one stained to show the nuclear pattern (Nissl preparation for cell bodies), the other stained to show fiber tracts (Weil preparation for myelin sheaths). The many different views of major structures, nuclear groups, tracts, and pathways give the student a three-dimensional picture of the structural organization of the human central nervous system. In addition, we have illustrated the major blood supply and venous drainage of the brain by means of radio-angiograms and diagrams.

In expanding this atlas to include more sections and different planes of section, we have made it more detailed and comprehensive than many introductory courses in neuroanatomy would require. In this case selections can be made to suit the level of the course. Our intent was to make the atlas useful to a wide range of students of the human nervous system—medical, dental, allied health professional, graduate, post-graduate, and any other curious student, whatever his or her level.

The Medical College of Pennsylvania
Philadelphia   S. J. D.

and

The State University of New York   M. M. F.
Stony Brook   M. M. D.

March 1974

THE GROSS BRAIN AND SPINAL CORD

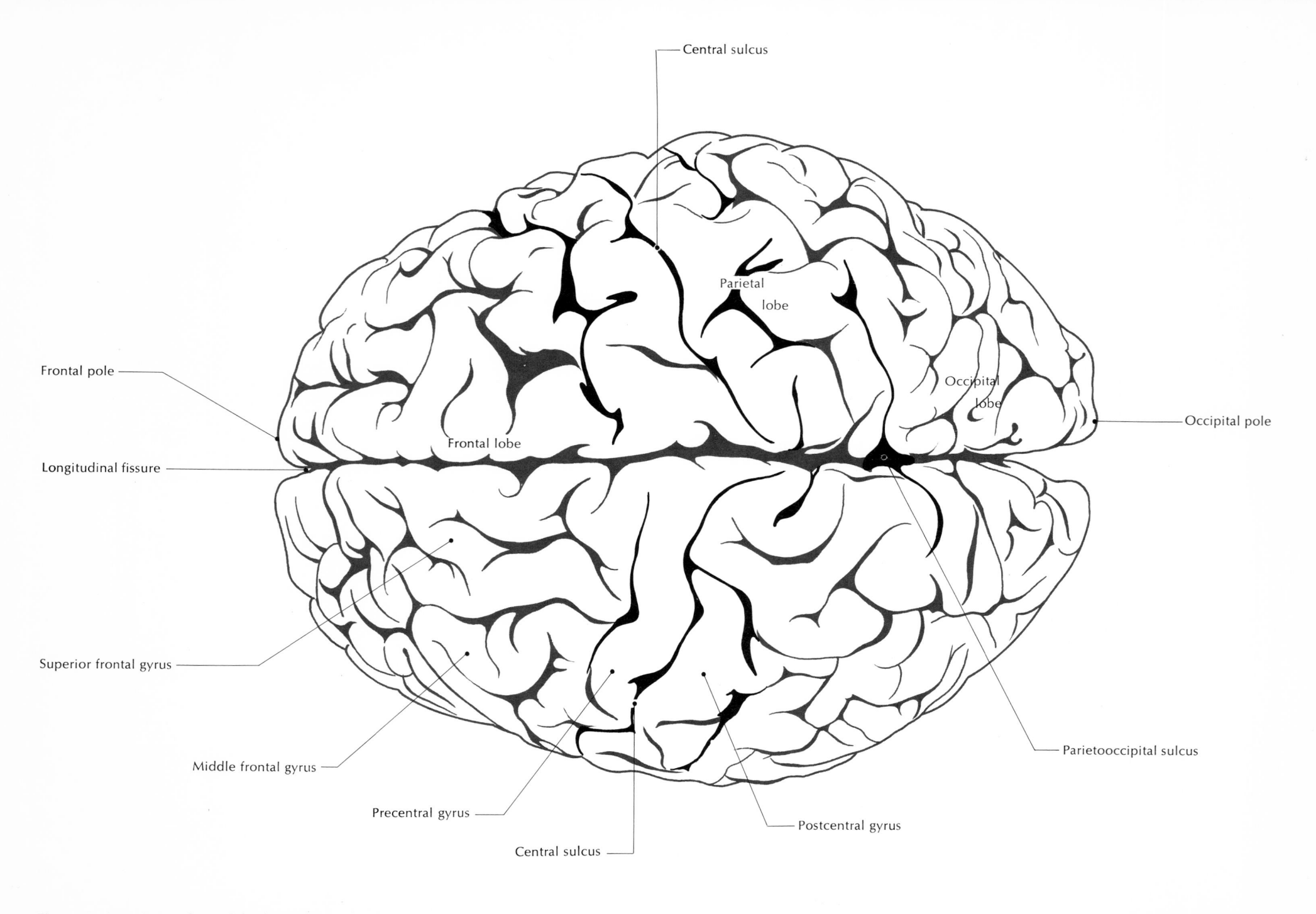

Central sulcus

Parietal
lobe

Occipital
lobe

Frontal pole

Occipital pole

Frontal lobe

Longitudinal fissure

Superior frontal gyrus

Parietooccipital sulcus

Middle frontal gyrus

Precentral gyrus

Postcentral gyrus

Central sulcus

Figure 1. Superior surface of the brain—actual size

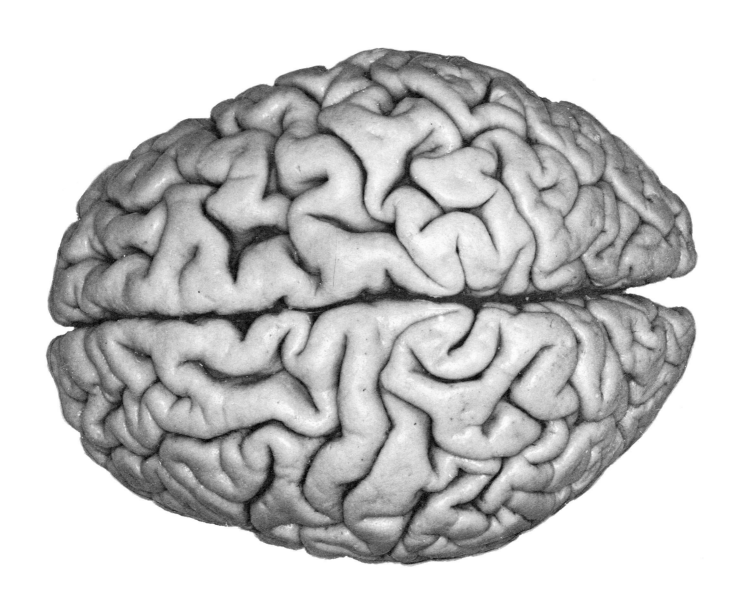

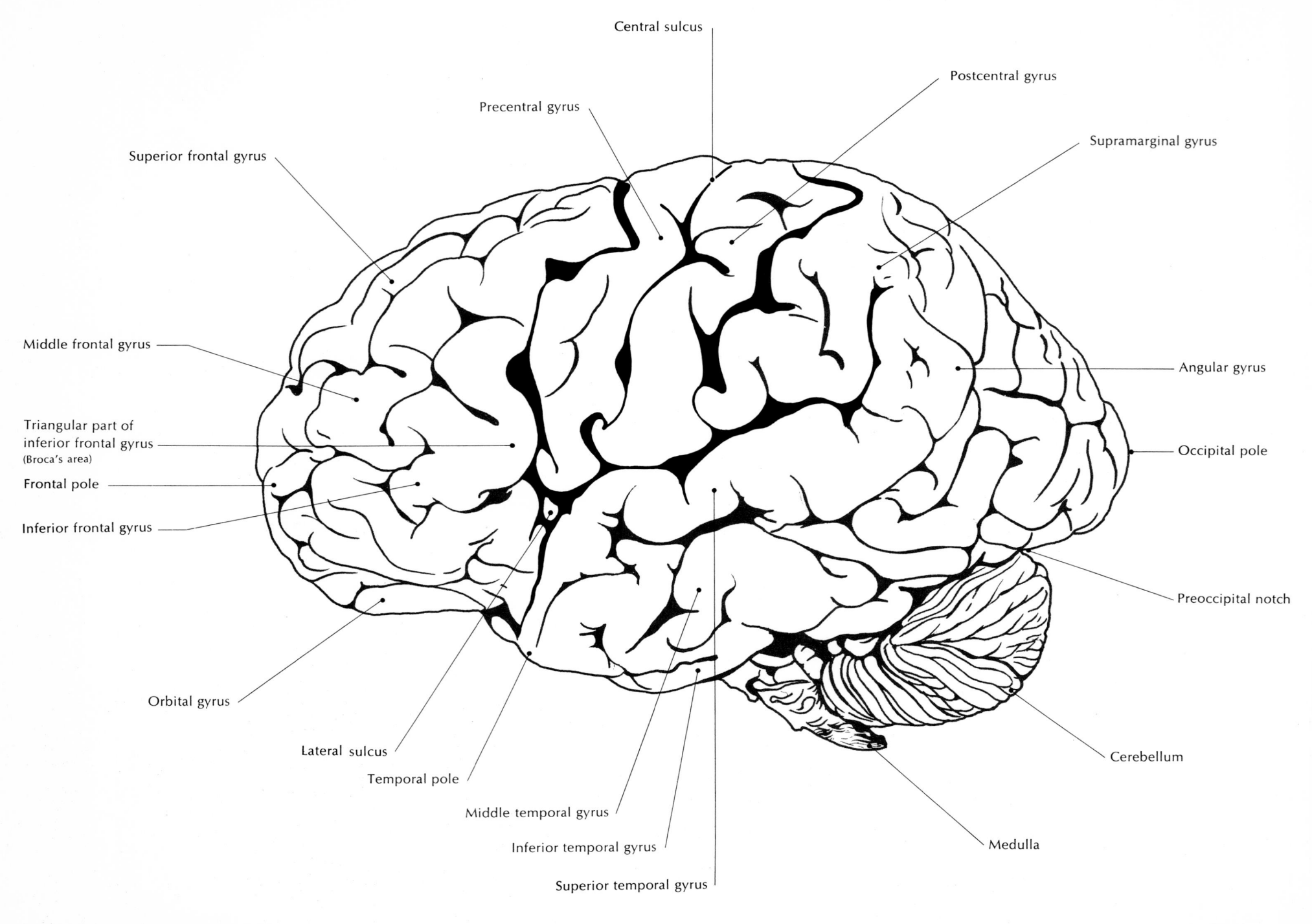

Central sulcus

Postcentral gyrus

Precentral gyrus

Supramarginal gyrus

Superior frontal gyrus

Middle frontal gyrus

Angular gyrus

Triangular part of
inferior frontal gyrus
(Broca's area)

Occipital pole

Frontal pole

Inferior frontal gyrus

Preoccipital notch

Orbital gyrus

Cerebellum

Lateral sulcus

Temporal pole

Middle temporal gyrus

Inferior temporal gyrus

Medulla

Superior temporal gyrus

Figure 2. Lateral surface of the brain—actual size

4

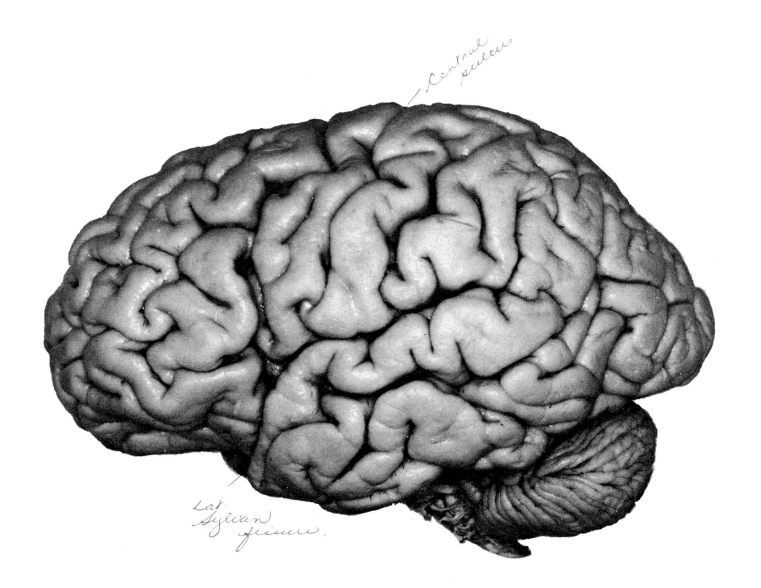

Central Sulcus

Lat. Sylvian fissure.

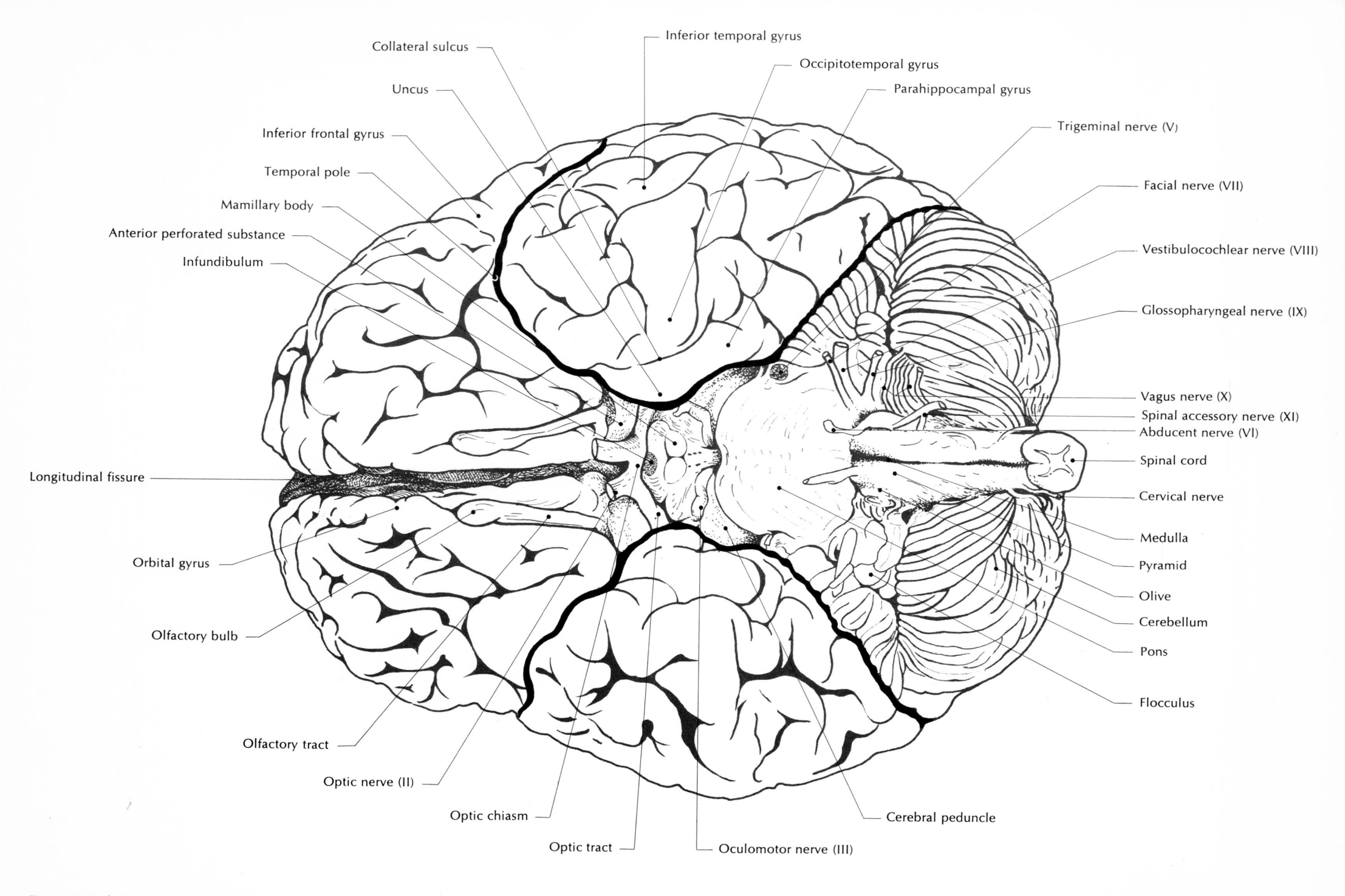

Figure 3. Inferior surface of the brain—actual size

6

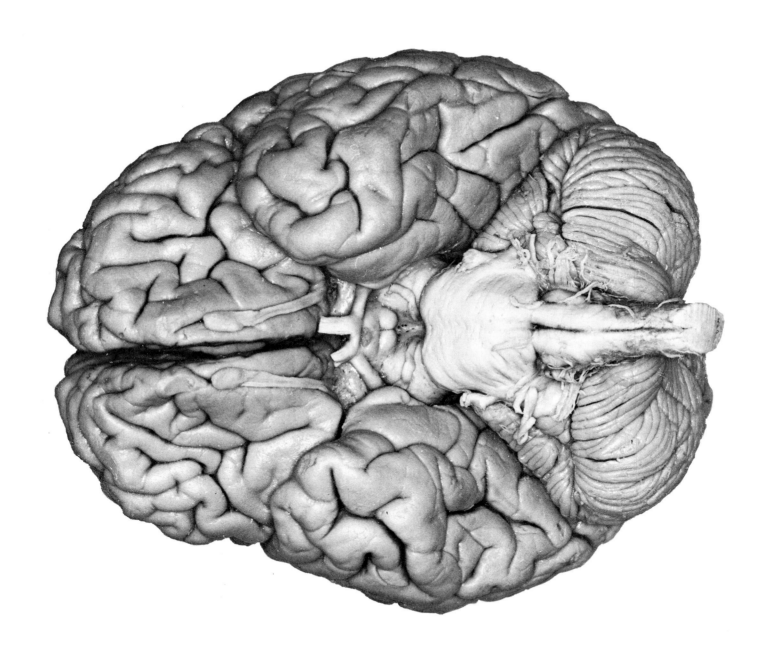

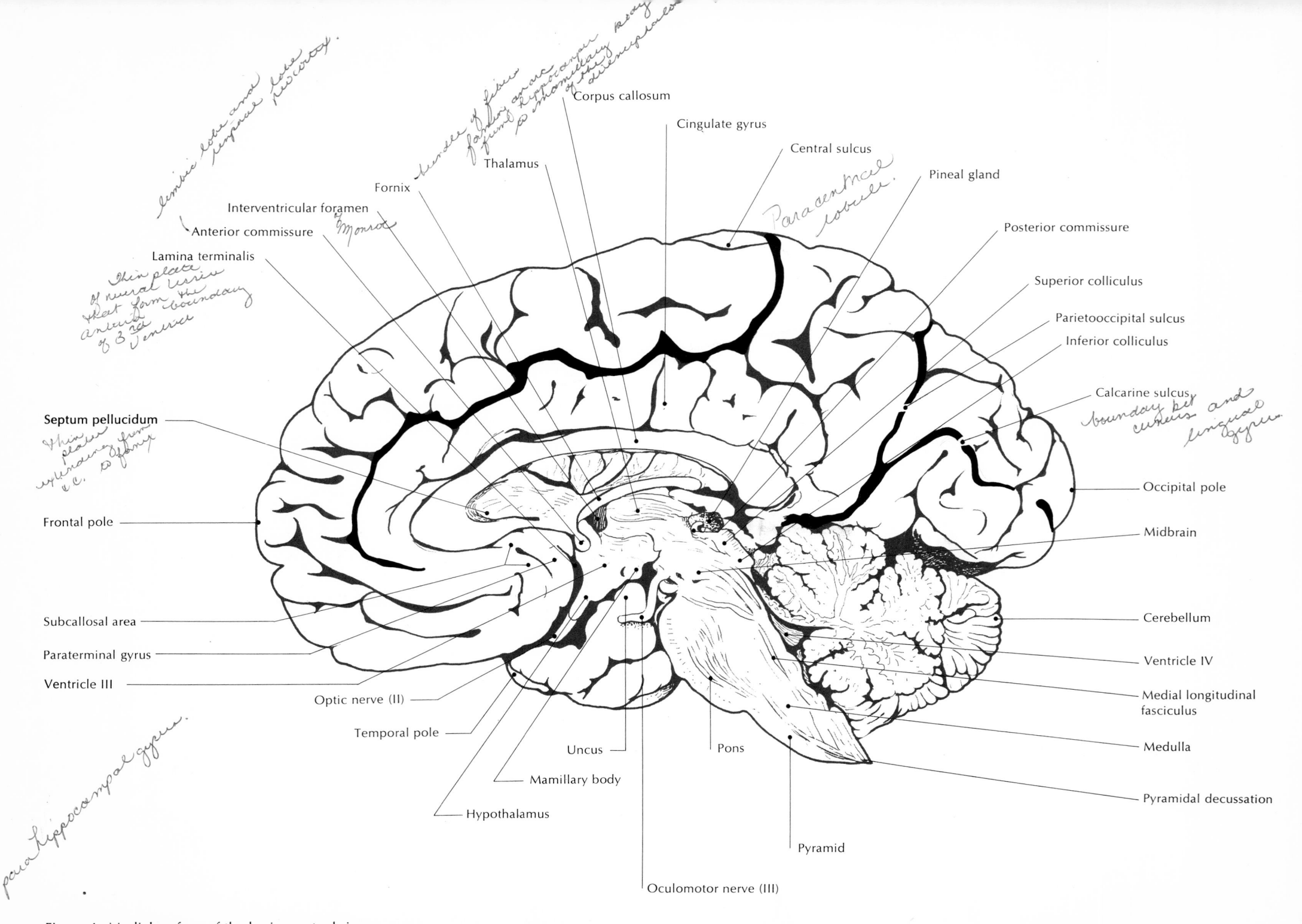

Corpus callosum

Cingulate gyrus

Central sulcus

Thalamus

Pineal gland

Fornix

Posterior commissure

Interventricular foramen

Anterior commissure

Superior colliculus

Lamina terminalis

Parietooccipital sulcus

Inferior colliculus

Septum pellucidum

Calcarine sulcus

Occipital pole

Frontal pole

Midbrain

Subcallosal area

Cerebellum

Paraterminal gyrus

Ventricle IV

Ventricle III

Medial longitudinal fasciculus

Optic nerve (II)

Temporal pole

Medulla

Uncus

Pons

Pyramidal decussation

Mamillary body

Hypothalamus

Pyramid

Oculomotor nerve (III)

Figure 4. Medial surface of the brain—actual size

8

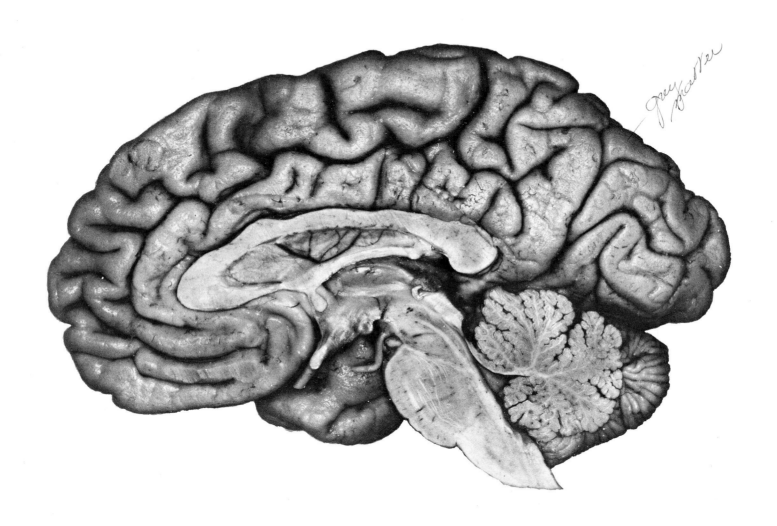

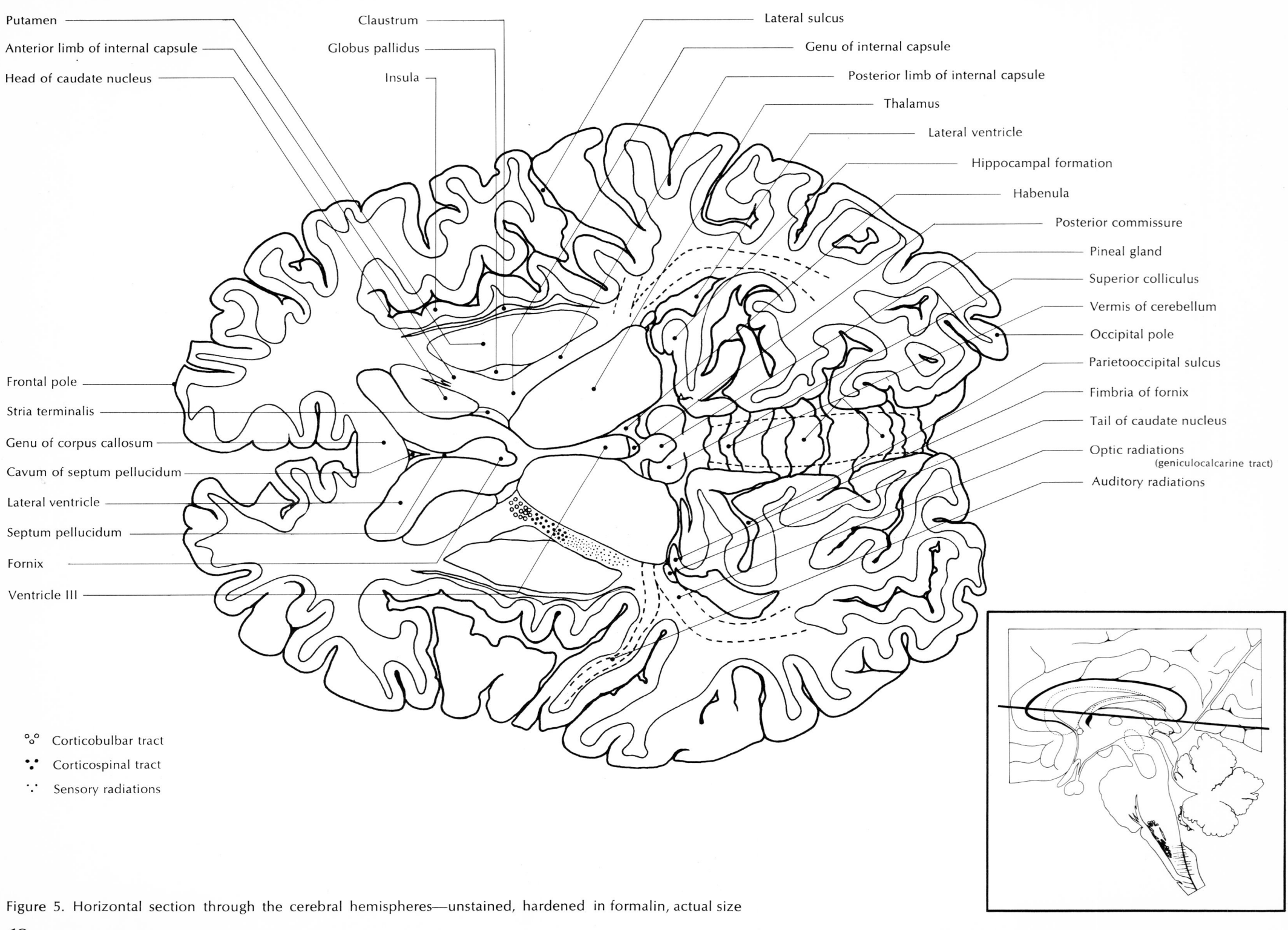

Putamen

Anterior limb of internal capsule

Head of caudate nucleus

Claustrum

Globus pallidus

Insula

Lateral sulcus

Genu of internal capsule

Posterior limb of internal capsule

Thalamus

Lateral ventricle

Hippocampal formation

Habenula

Posterior commissure

Pineal gland

Superior colliculus

Vermis of cerebellum

Occipital pole

Parietooccipital sulcus

Fimbria of fornix

Tail of caudate nucleus

Optic radiations
(geniculocalcarine tract)

Auditory radiations

Frontal pole

Stria terminalis

Genu of corpus callosum

Cavum of septum pellucidum

Lateral ventricle

Septum pellucidum

Fornix

Ventricle III

○°○ Corticobulbar tract

•∴• Corticospinal tract

∴ Sensory radiations

Figure 5. Horizontal section through the cerebral hemispheres—unstained, hardened in formalin, actual size

10

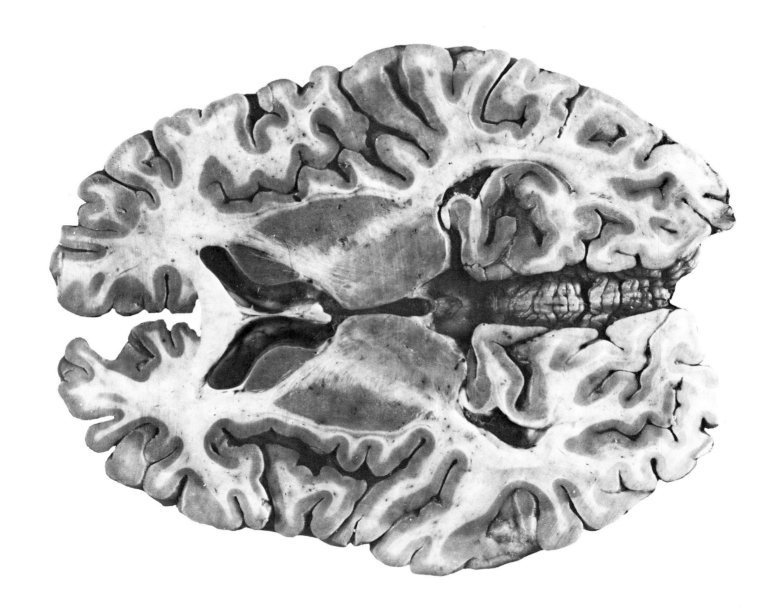

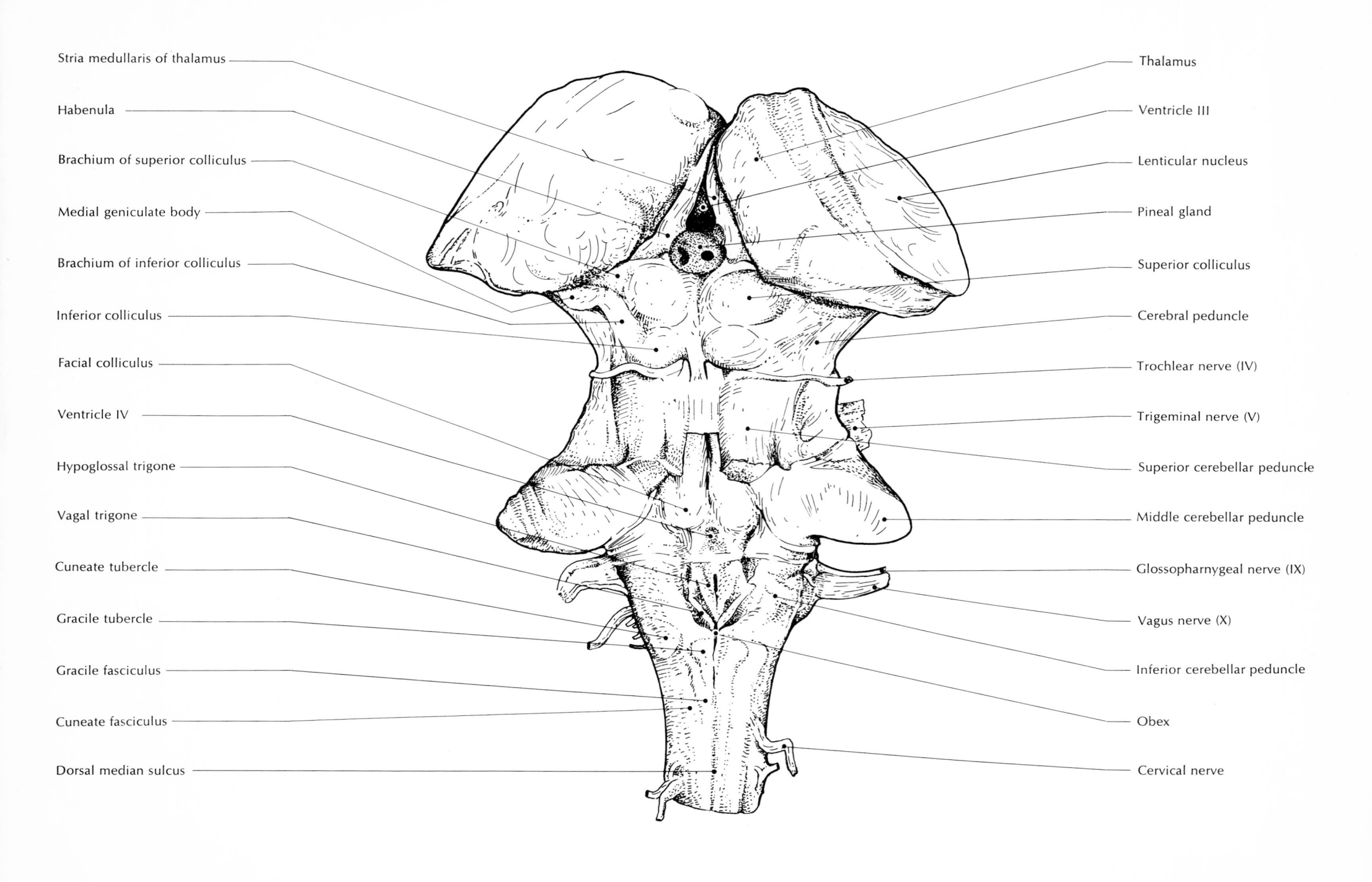

Stria medullaris of thalamus

Habenula

Brachium of superior colliculus

Medial geniculate body

Brachium of inferior colliculus

Inferior colliculus

Facial colliculus

Ventricle IV

Hypoglossal trigone

Vagal trigone

Cuneate tubercle

Gracile tubercle

Gracile fasciculus

Cuneate fasciculus

Dorsal median sulcus

Thalamus

Ventricle III

Lenticular nucleus

Pineal gland

Superior colliculus

Cerebral peduncle

Trochlear nerve (IV)

Trigeminal nerve (V)

Superior cerebellar peduncle

Middle cerebellar peduncle

Glossopharnygeal nerve (IX)

Vagus nerve (X)

Inferior cerebellar peduncle

Obex

Cervical nerve

Figure 6. Dorsal surface of the brain stem—1.5X

12

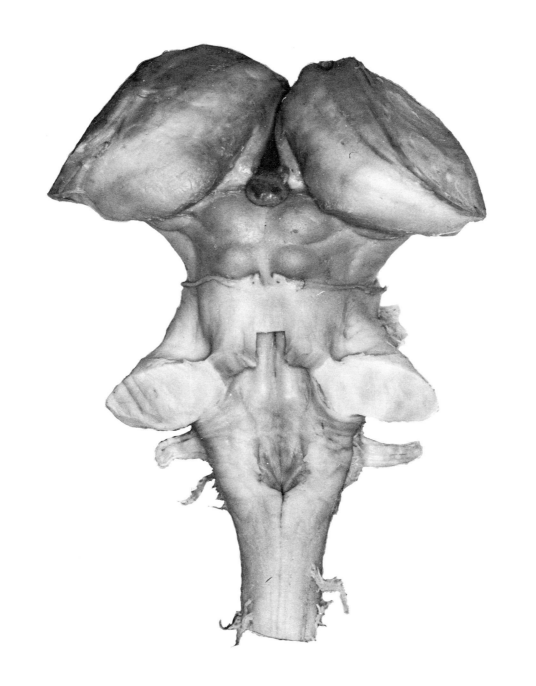

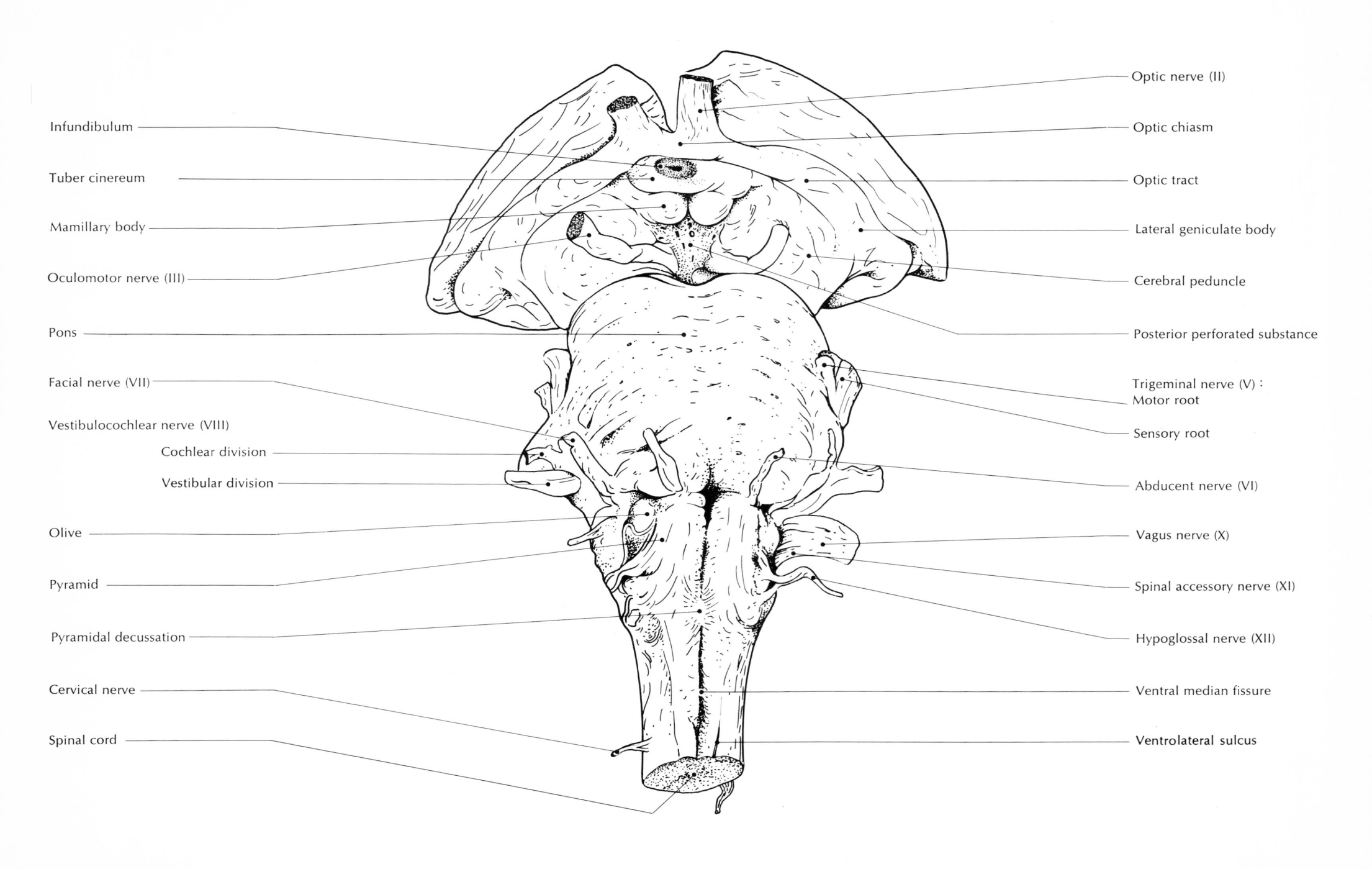

Optic nerve (II)

Infundibulum

Optic chiasm

Tuber cinereum

Optic tract

Mamillary body

Lateral geniculate body

Oculomotor nerve (III)

Cerebral peduncle

Pons

Posterior perforated substance

Facial nerve (VII)

Trigeminal nerve (V) :
Motor root

Vestibulocochlear nerve (VIII)

Sensory root

Cochlear division

Vestibular division

Abducent nerve (VI)

Olive

Vagus nerve (X)

Pyramid

Spinal accessory nerve (XI)

Pyramidal decussation

Hypoglossal nerve (XII)

Cervical nerve

Ventral median fissure

Spinal cord

Ventrolateral sulcus

Figure 7. Ventral surface of the brain stem—1.5X

14

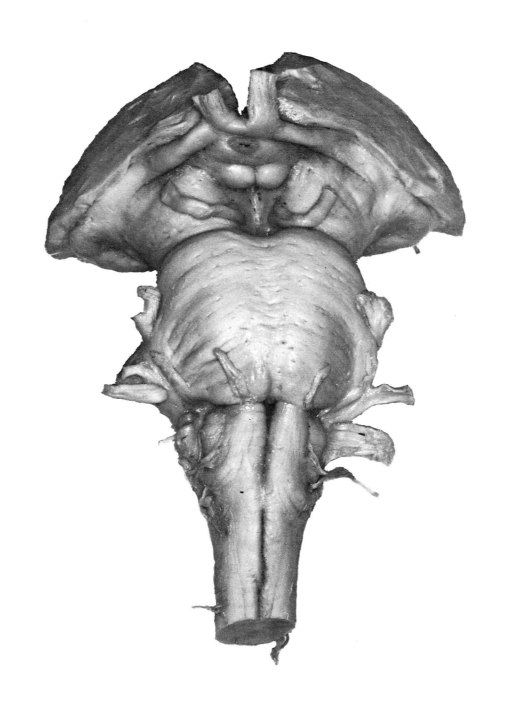

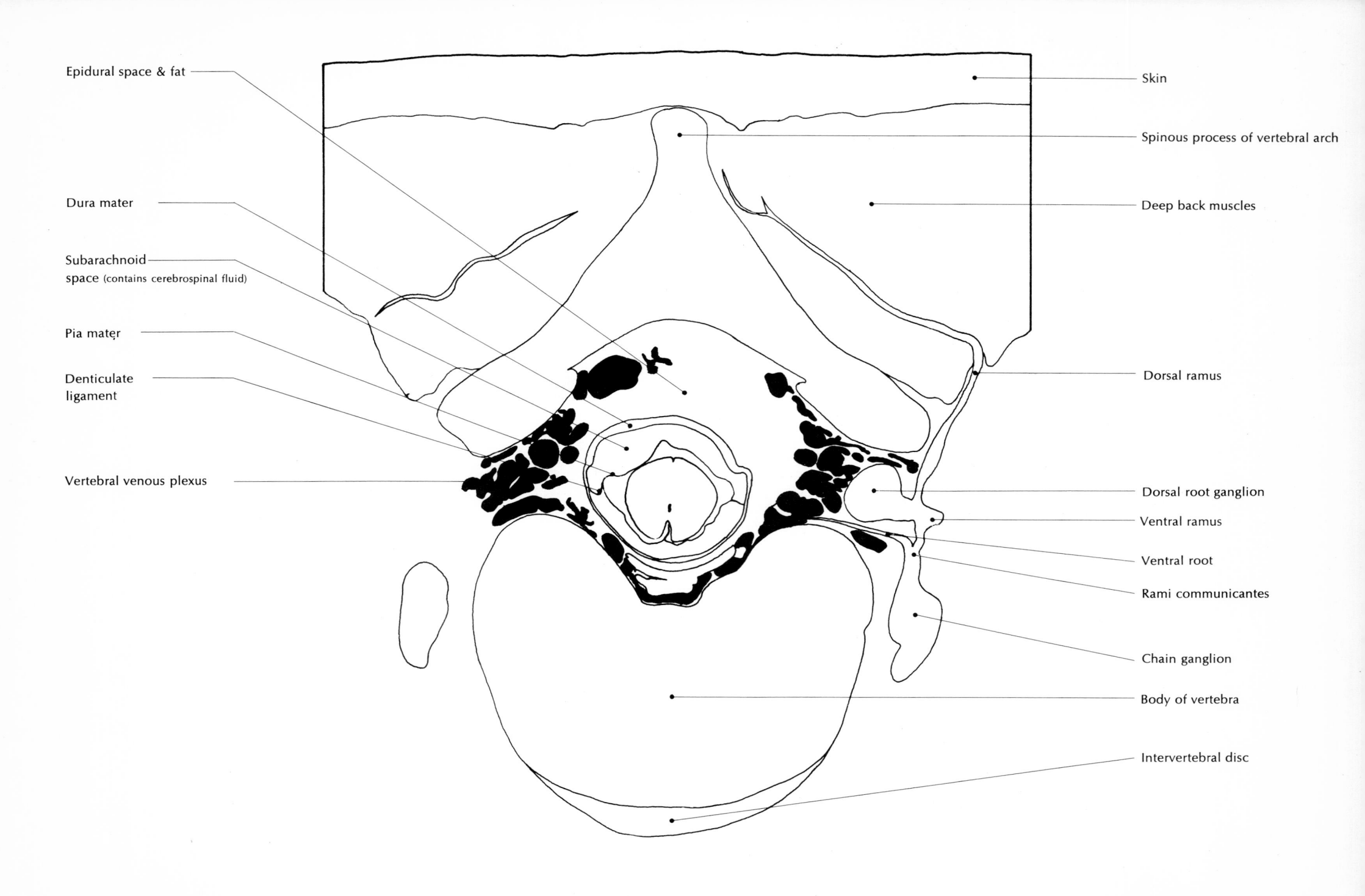

Epidural space & fat

Dura mater

Subarachnoid space (contains cerebrospinal fluid)

Pia mater

Denticulate ligament

Vertebral venous plexus

Skin

Spinous process of vertebral arch

Deep back muscles

Dorsal ramus

Dorsal root ganglion

Ventral ramus

Ventral root

Rami communicantes

Chain ganglion

Body of vertebra

Intervertebral disc

Figure 8. Transverse section of the thoracic spinal cord *in situ,* newborn—Hematoxylin and Eosin, 8.7X

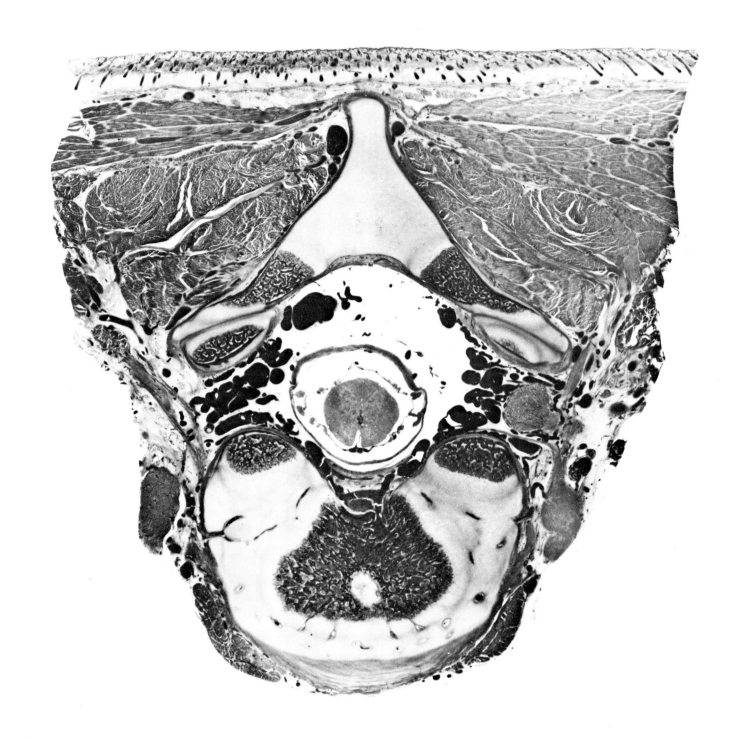

TRANSVERSE SECTIONS OF THE SPINAL CORD

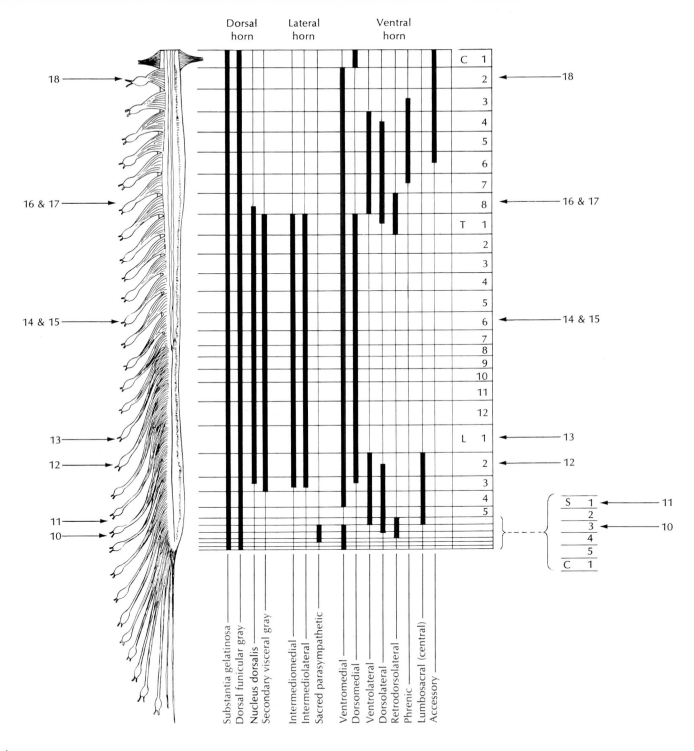

Figure 9. Nuclear columns of the spinal cord

19

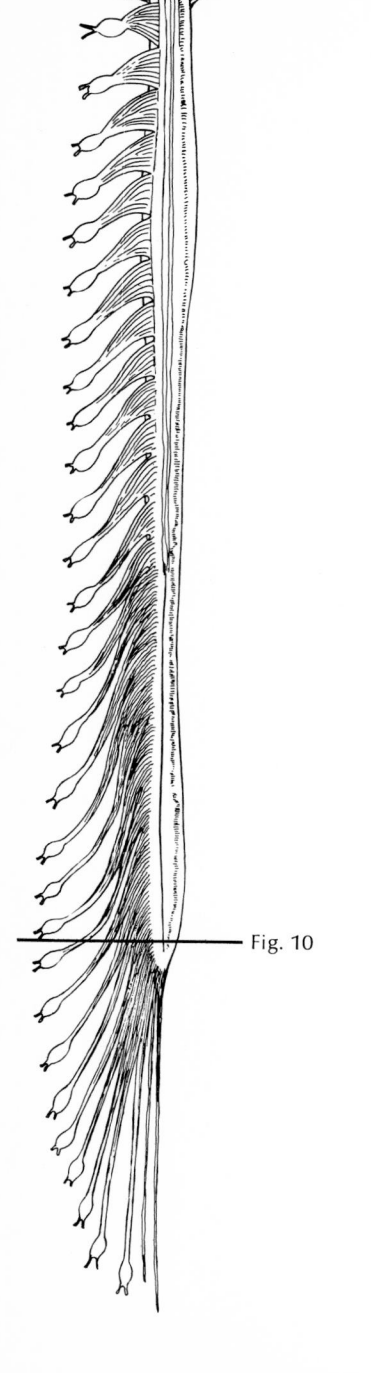

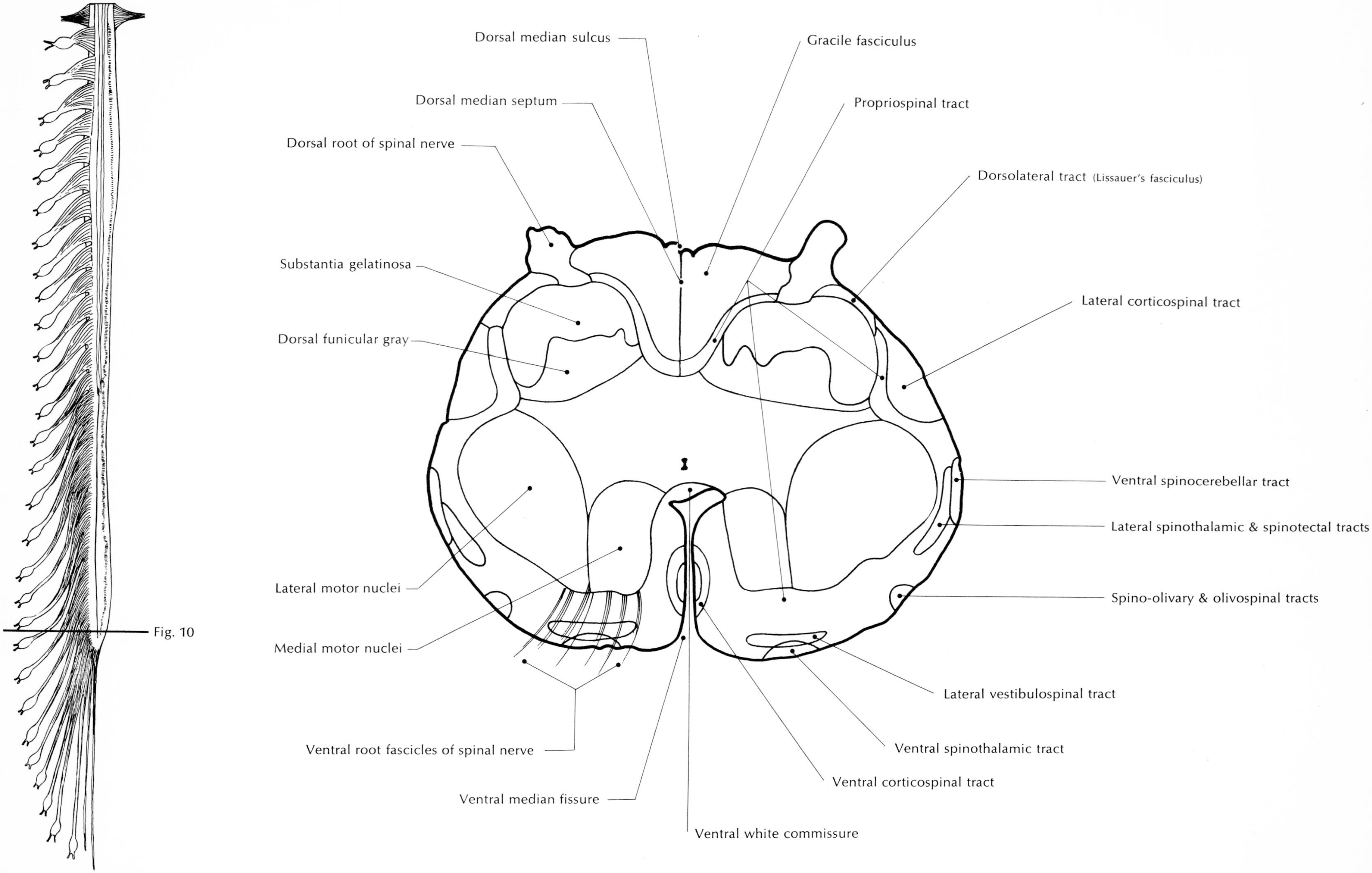

Dorsal median sulcus —

Gracile fasciculus

Dorsal median septum —

Propriospinal tract

Dorsal root of spinal nerve —

Dorsolateral tract (Lissauer's fasciculus)

Substantia gelatinosa —

Lateral corticospinal tract

Dorsal funicular gray —

Ventral spinocerebellar tract

Lateral spinothalamic & spinotectal tracts

Spino-olivary & olivospinal tracts

Lateral motor nuclei —

Medial motor nuclei —

Lateral vestibulospinal tract

Ventral root fascicles of spinal nerve —

Ventral spinothalamic tract

Ventral corticospinal tract

Ventral median fissure —

Ventral white commissure

Fig. 10

Figure 10. Sacral cord (S3)—Weil, 18X

20

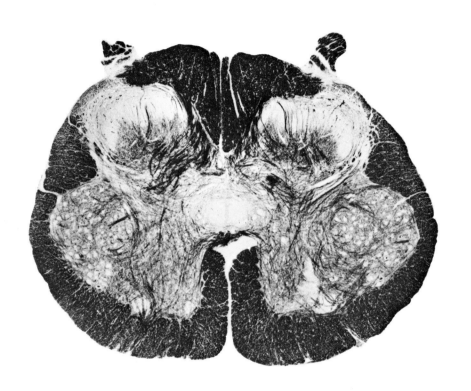

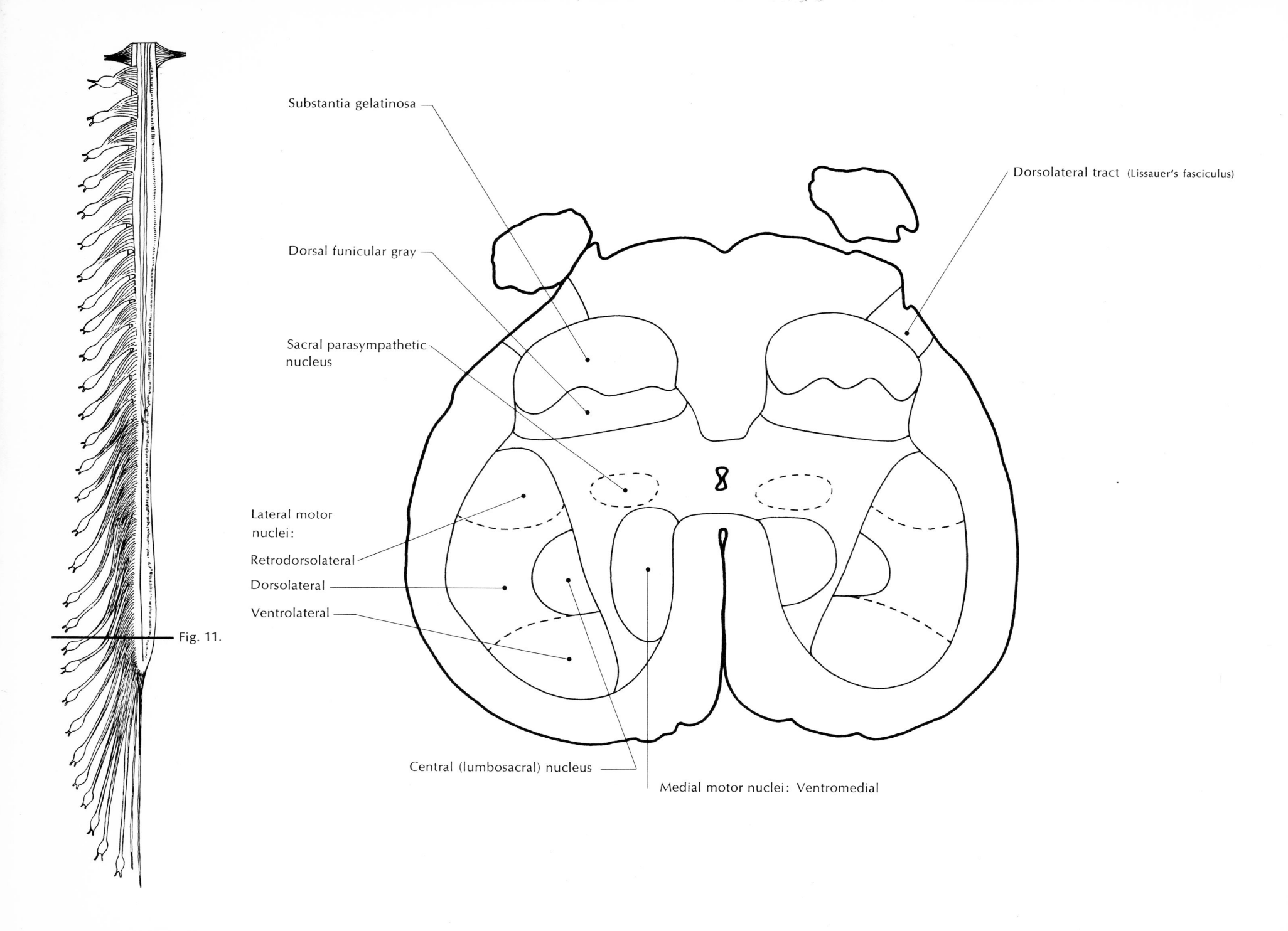

Substantia gelatinosa

Dorsal funicular gray

Sacral parasympathetic nucleus

Dorsolateral tract (Lissauer's fasciculus)

Lateral motor nuclei:

Retrodorsolateral

Dorsolateral

Ventrolateral

Fig. 11.

Central (lumbosacral) nucleus

Medial motor nuclei: Ventromedial

Figure 11. Sacral cord (S1)—Nissl, 18X

22

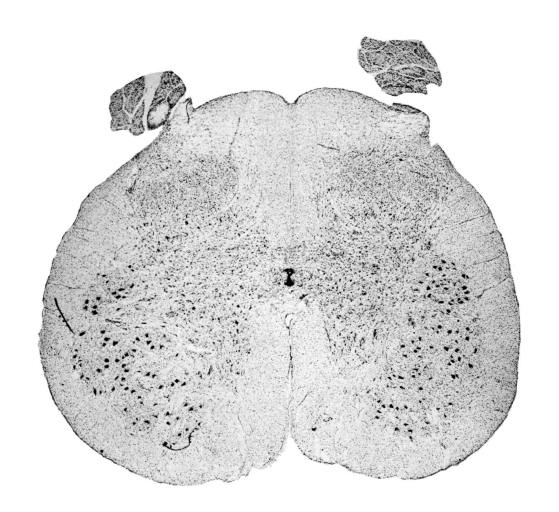

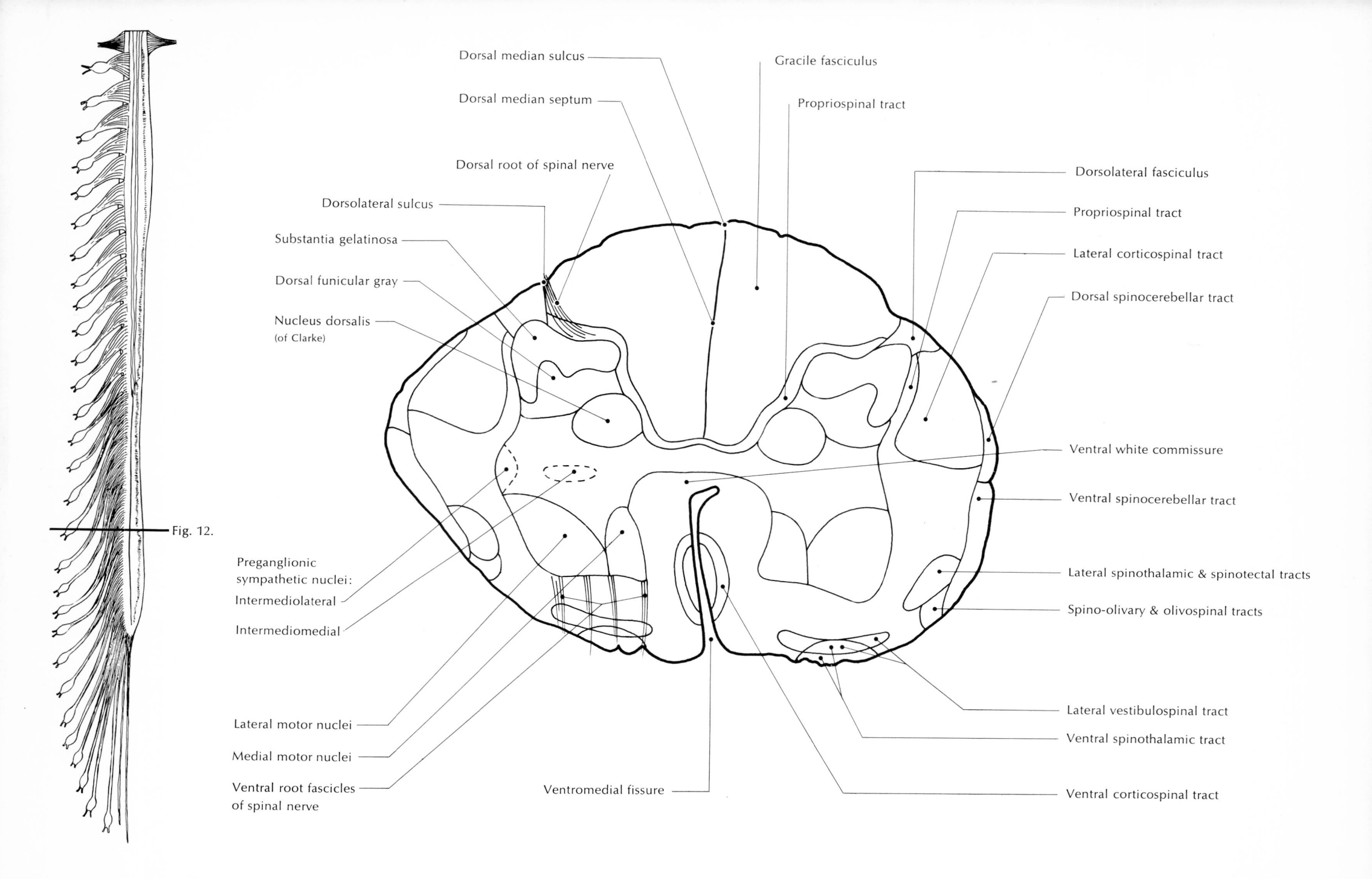

Dorsal median sulcus

Dorsal median septum

Dorsal root of spinal nerve

Gracile fasciculus

Propriospinal tract

Dorsolateral sulcus

Substantia gelatinosa

Dorsal funicular gray

Nucleus dorsalis
(of Clarke)

Dorsolateral fasciculus

Propriospinal tract

Lateral corticospinal tract

Dorsal spinocerebellar tract

Ventral white commissure

Ventral spinocerebellar tract

Preganglionic
sympathetic nuclei:

Intermediolateral

Intermediomedial

Lateral spinothalamic & spinotectal tracts

Spino-olivary & olivospinal tracts

Lateral motor nuclei

Medial motor nuclei

Ventral root fascicles
of spinal nerve

Ventromedial fissure

Lateral vestibulospinal tract

Ventral spinothalamic tract

Ventral corticospinal tract

Fig. 12.

Figure 12. Lumbar cord (L2)—Weil, 18X

24

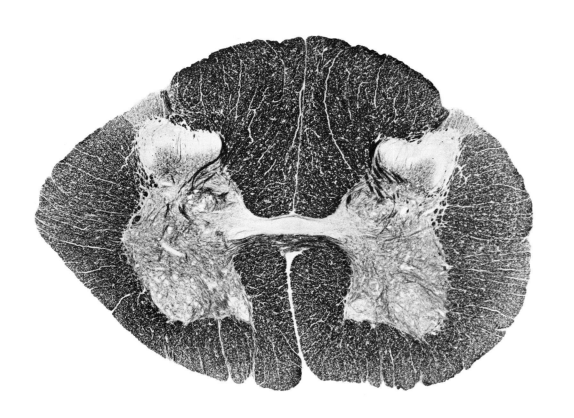

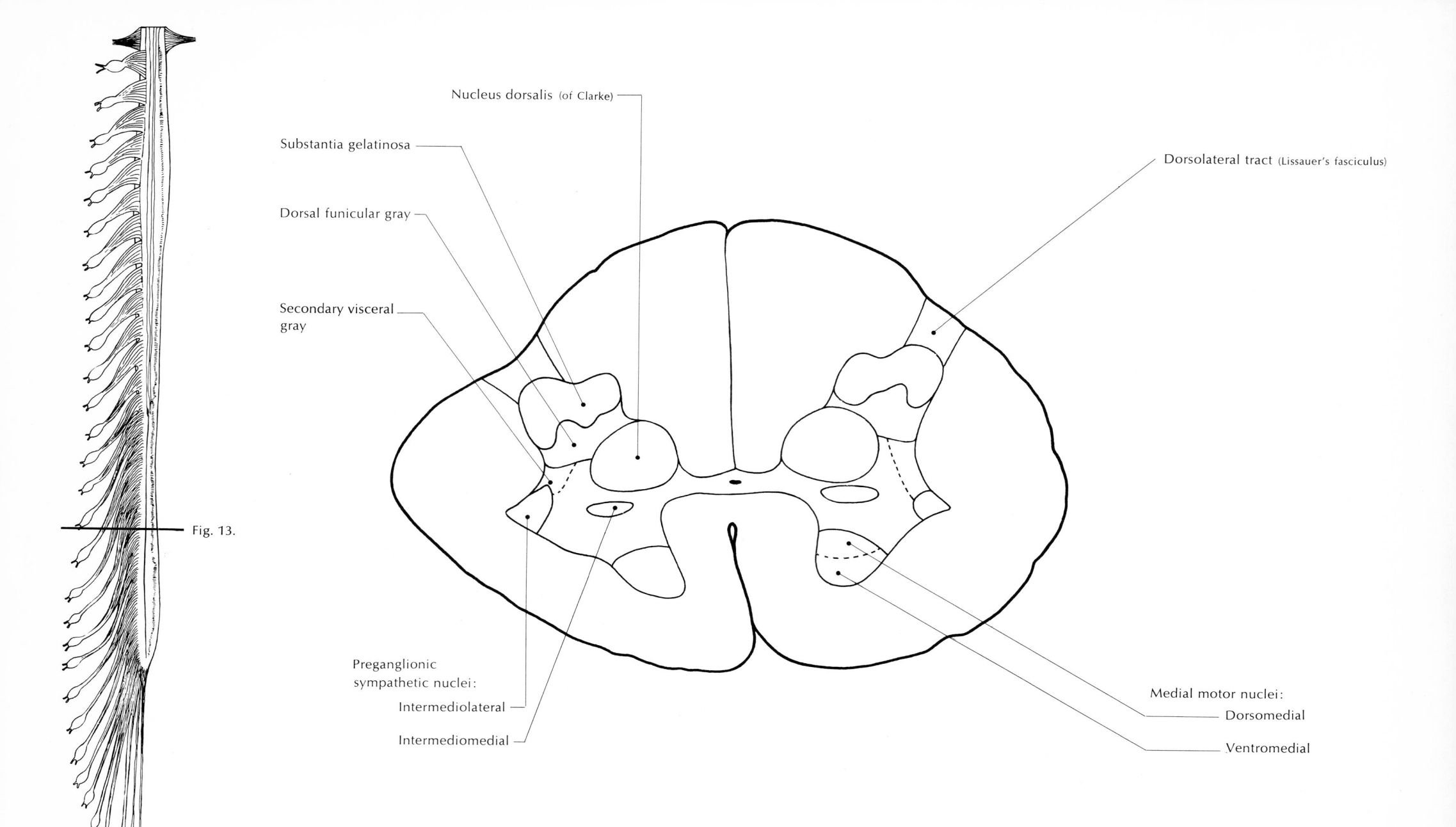

Nucleus dorsalis (of Clarke)

Substantia gelatinosa

Dorsolateral tract (Lissauer's fasciculus)

Dorsal funicular gray

Secondary visceral gray

Preganglionic
sympathetic nuclei:

Intermediolateral

Intermediomedial

Medial motor nuclei:

Dorsomedial

Ventromedial

Fig. 13.

Figure 13. Lumbar cord (L1)—Nissl, 18X

26

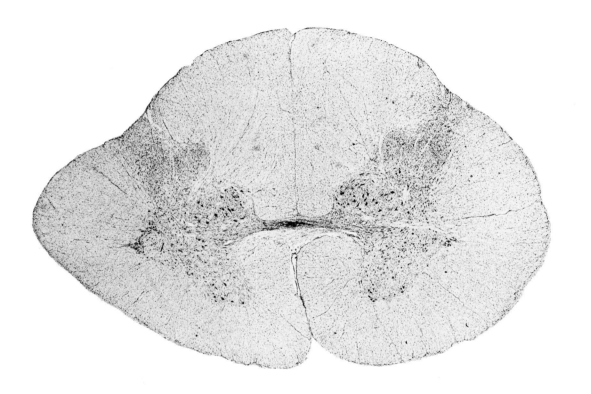

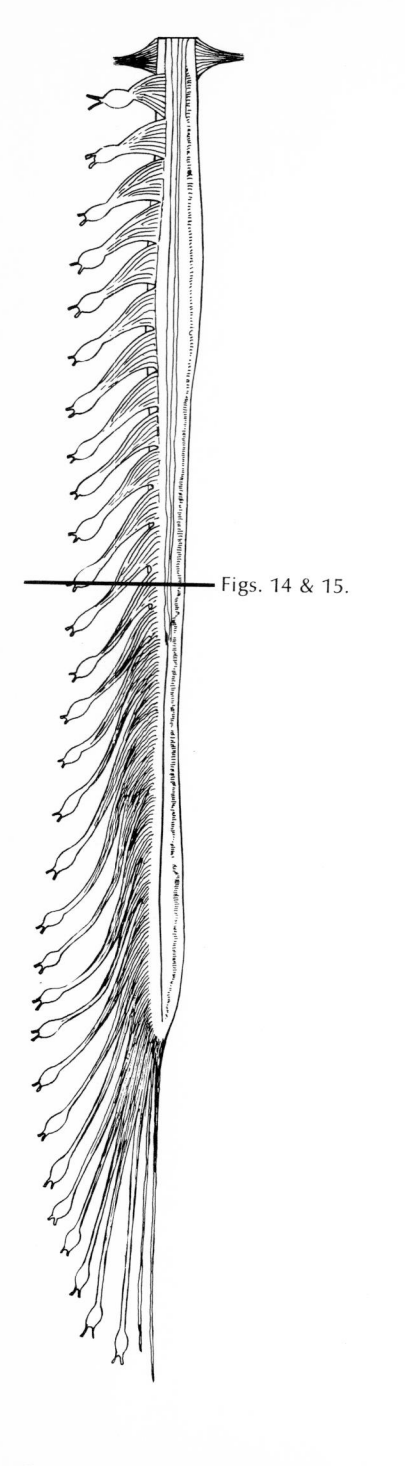

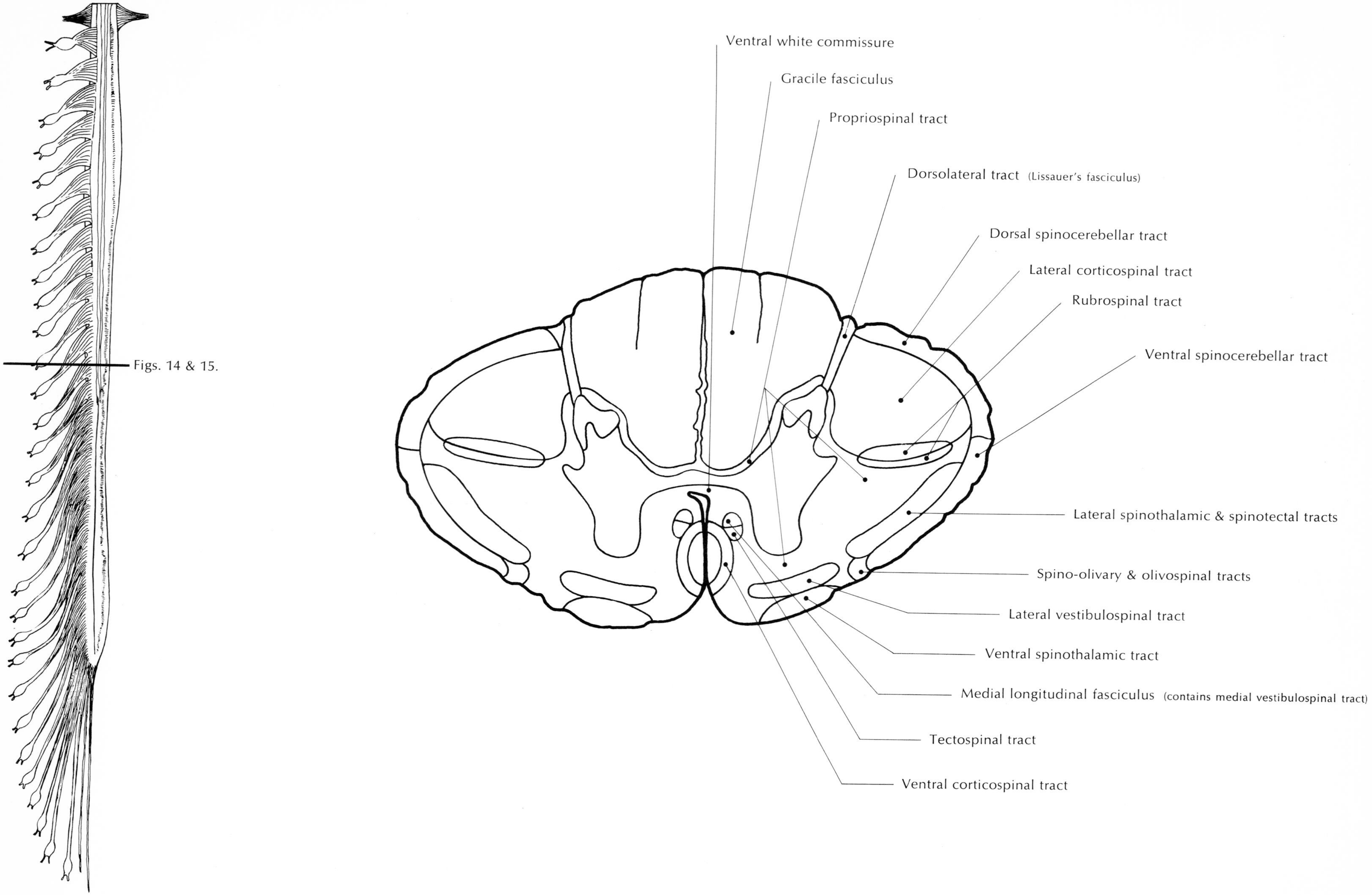

Ventral white commissure

Gracile fasciculus

Propriospinal tract

Dorsolateral tract (Lissauer's fasciculus)

Dorsal spinocerebellar tract

Lateral corticospinal tract

Rubrospinal tract

Ventral spinocerebellar tract

Lateral spinothalamic & spinotectal tracts

Spino-olivary & olivospinal tracts

Lateral vestibulospinal tract

Ventral spinothalamic tract

Medial longitudinal fasciculus (contains medial vestibulospinal tract)

Tectospinal tract

Ventral corticospinal tract

Figs. 14 & 15.

Figure 14. Thoracic cord (T6)—Weil, 18X

28

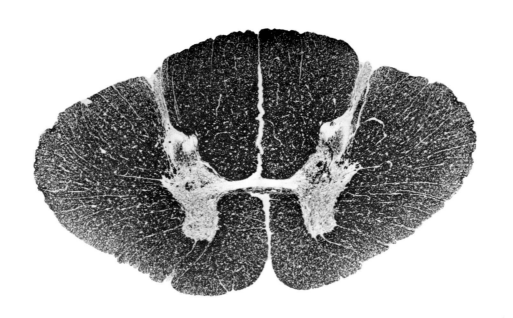

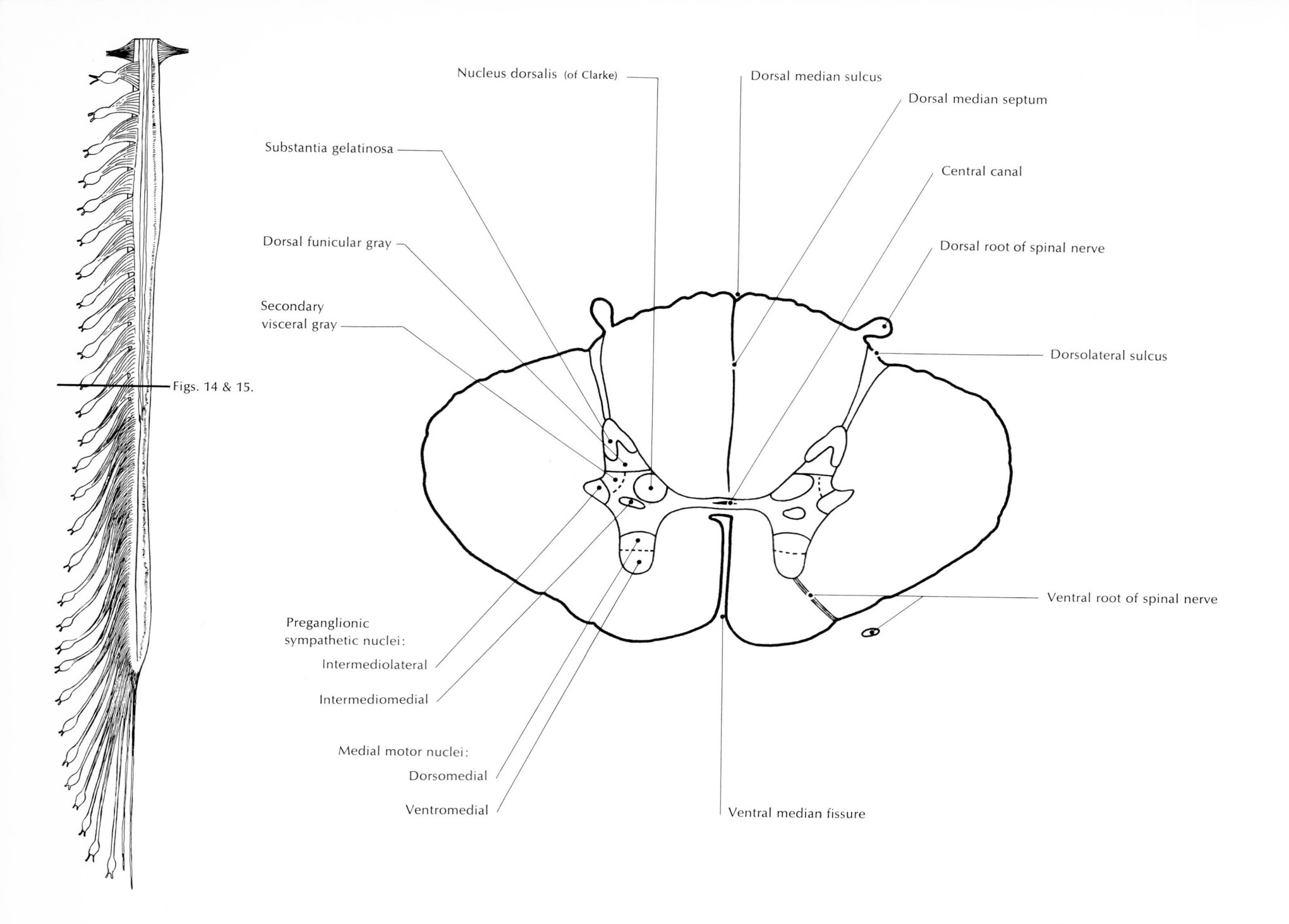

Nucleus dorsalis (of Clarke)

Dorsal median sulcus

Dorsal median septum

Substantia gelatinosa

Central canal

Dorsal funicular gray

Dorsal root of spinal nerve

Secondary visceral gray

Dorsolateral sulcus

Figs. 14 & 15.

Ventral root of spinal nerve

Preganglionic sympathetic nuclei:

Intermediolateral

Intermediomedial

Medial motor nuclei:

Dorsomedial

Ventromedial

Ventral median fissure

Figure 15. Thoracic cord (T6)—Nissl, 18X

30

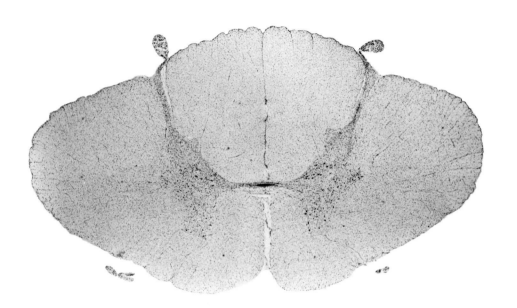

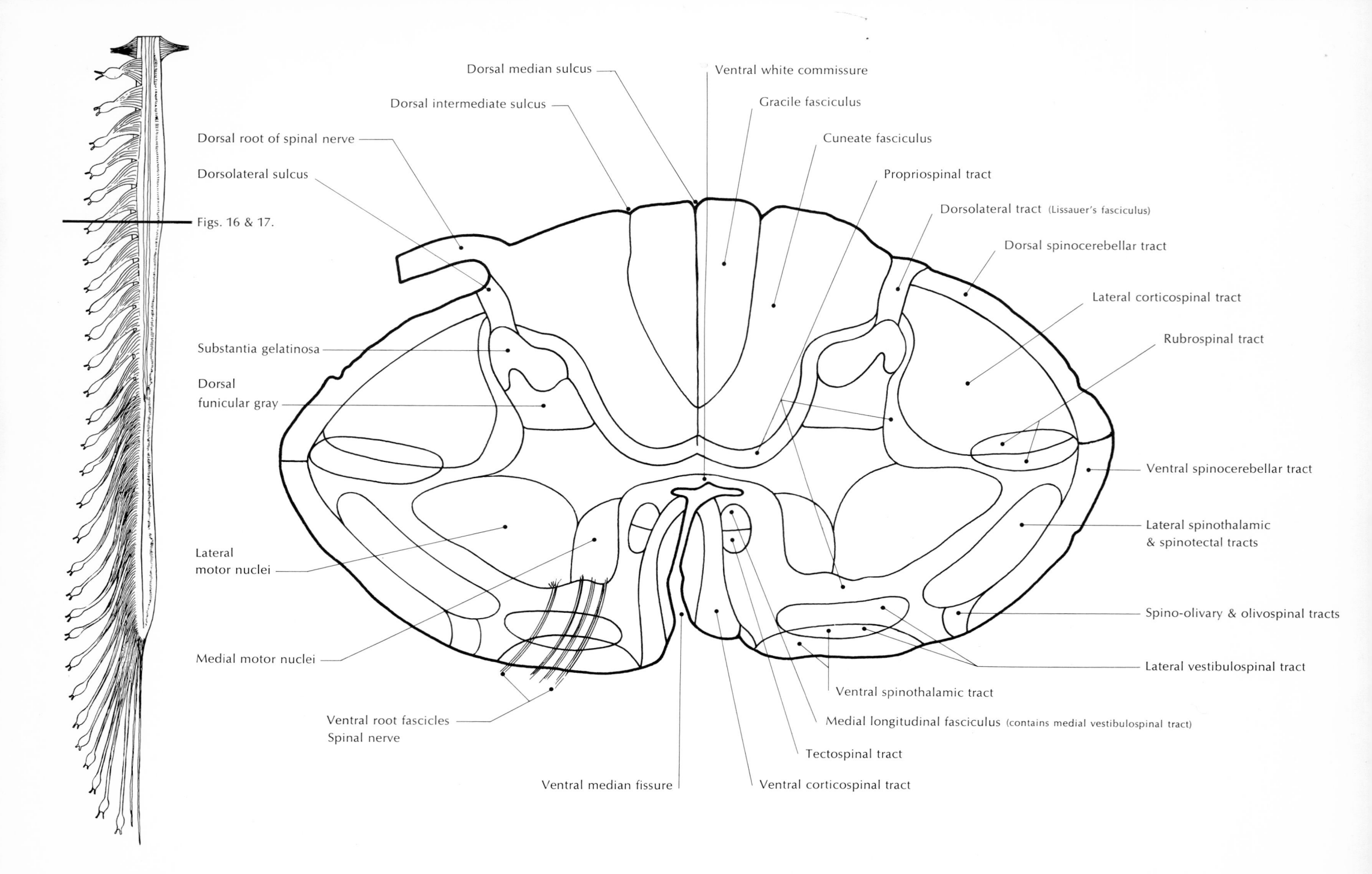

Dorsal median sulcus

Ventral white commissure

Dorsal intermediate sulcus

Gracile fasciculus

Dorsal root of spinal nerve

Cuneate fasciculus

Dorsolateral sulcus

Propriospinal tract

Figs. 16 & 17.

Dorsolateral tract (Lissauer's fasciculus)

Dorsal spinocerebellar tract

Substantia gelatinosa

Lateral corticospinal tract

Dorsal funicular gray

Rubrospinal tract

Lateral motor nuclei

Ventral spinocerebellar tract

Medial motor nuclei

Lateral spinothalamic & spinotectal tracts

Spino-olivary & olivospinal tracts

Lateral vestibulospinal tract

Ventral root fascicles Spinal nerve

Ventral spinothalamic tract

Medial longitudinal fasciculus (contains medial vestibulospinal tract)

Tectospinal tract

Ventral median fissure

Ventral corticospinal tract

Figure 16. Cervical cord enlargement (C8)—Weil, 18X

32

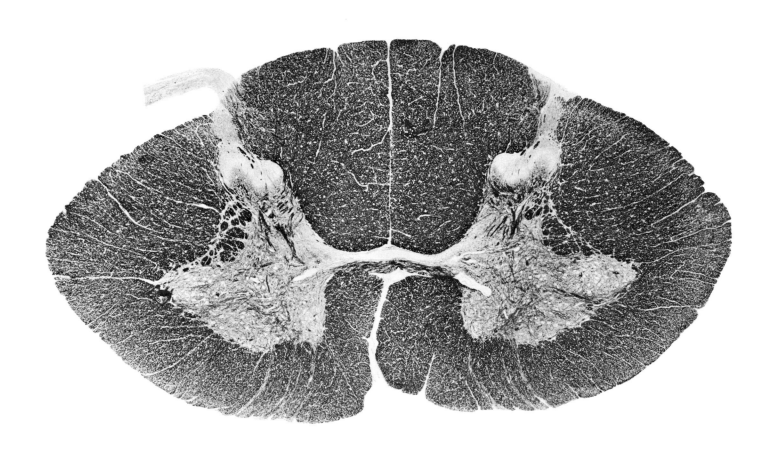

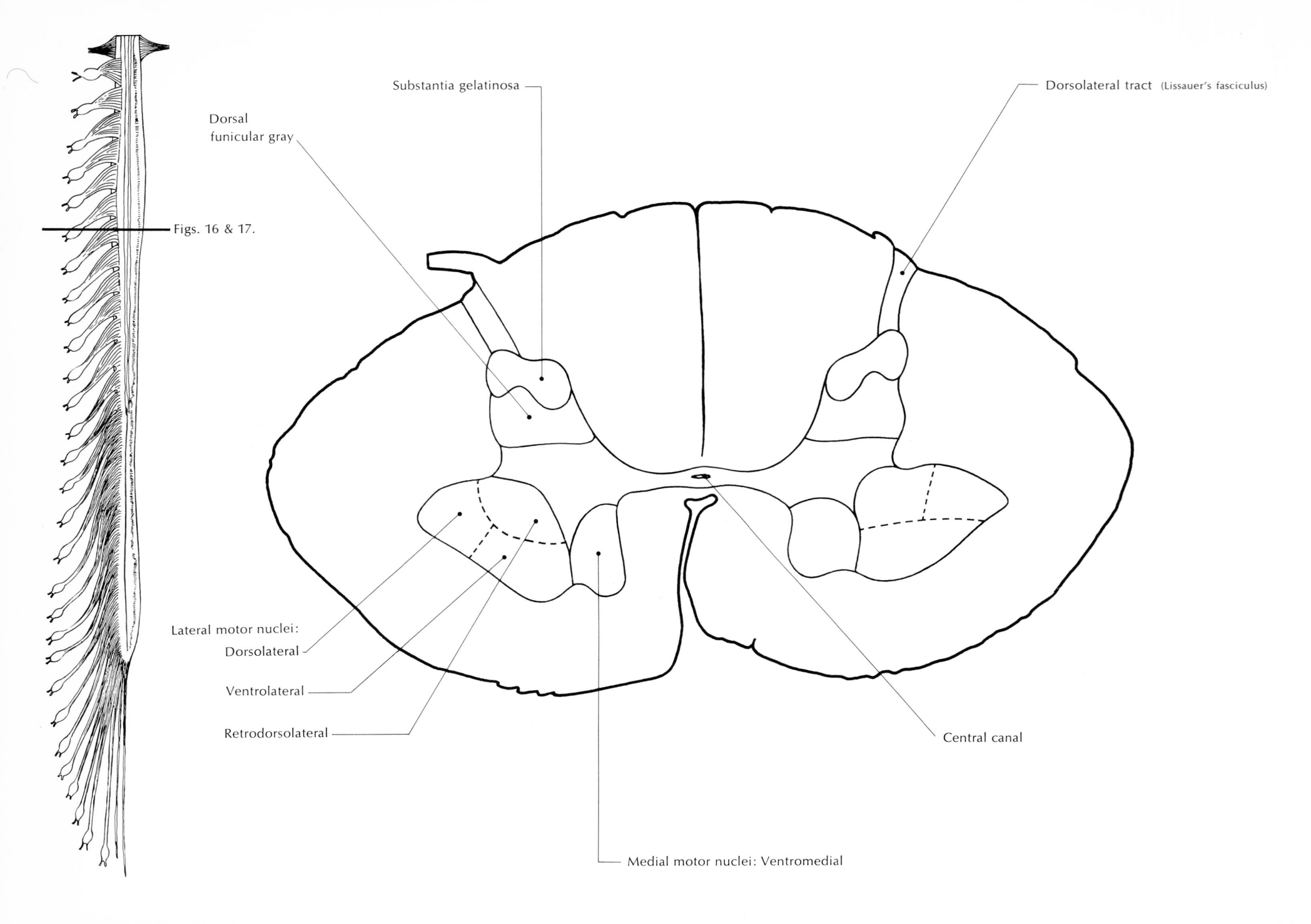

Substantia gelatinosa

Dorsolateral tract (Lissauer's fasciculus)

Dorsal funicular gray

Figs. 16 & 17.

Lateral motor nuclei:

Dorsolateral

Ventrolateral

Retrodorsolateral

Central canal

Medial motor nuclei: Ventromedial

Figure 17. Cervical cord enlargement (C8)—Nissl, 18X

34

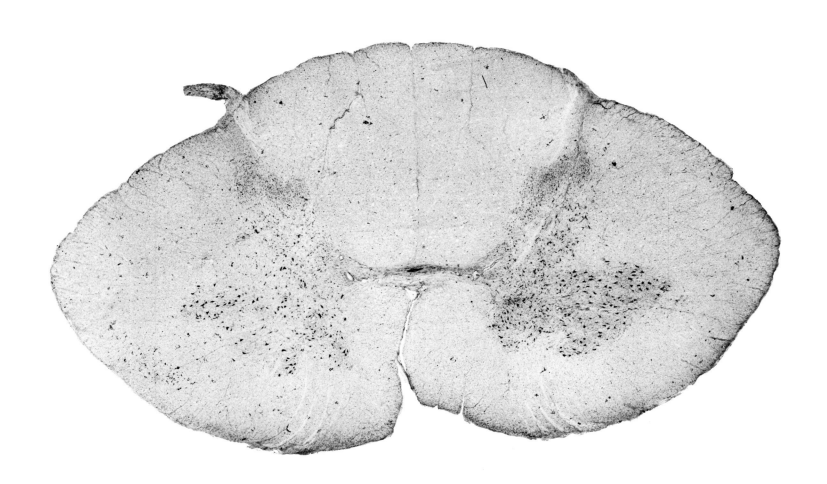

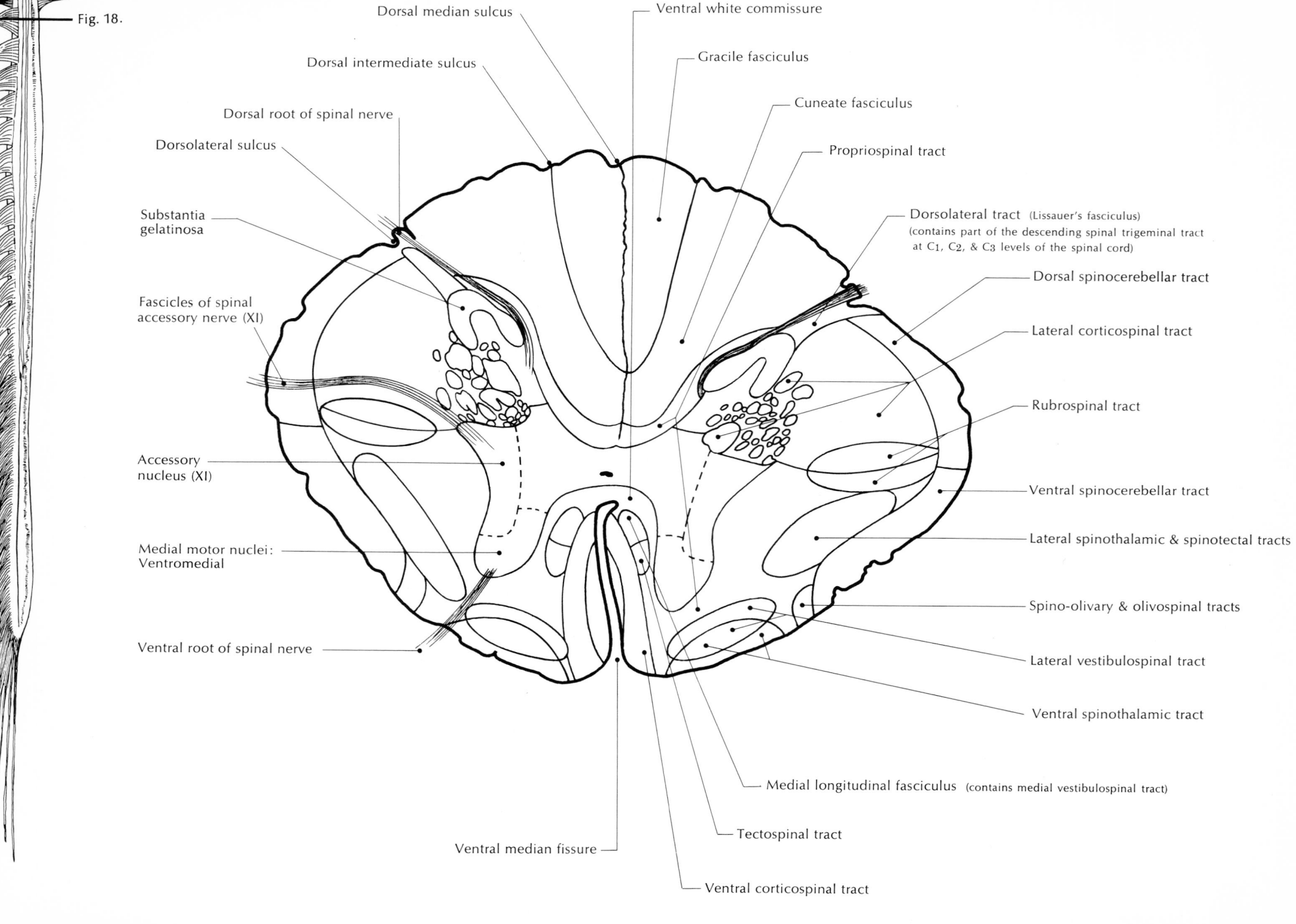

Fig. 18.

Dorsal median sulcus

Ventral white commissure

Gracile fasciculus

Dorsal intermediate sulcus

Cuneate fasciculus

Dorsal root of spinal nerve

Propriospinal tract

Dorsolateral sulcus

Dorsolateral tract (Lissauer's fasciculus)
(contains part of the descending spinal trigeminal tract
at C₁, C₂, & C₃ levels of the spinal cord)

Substantia
gelatinosa

Dorsal spinocerebellar tract

Fascicles of spinal
accessory nerve (XI)

Lateral corticospinal tract

Rubrospinal tract

Accessory
nucleus (XI)

Ventral spinocerebellar tract

Medial motor nuclei:
Ventromedial

Lateral spinothalamic & spinotectal tracts

Spino-olivary & olivospinal tracts

Ventral root of spinal nerve

Lateral vestibulospinal tract

Ventral spinothalamic tract

Medial longitudinal fasciculus (contains medial vestibulospinal tract)

Tectospinal tract

Ventral median fissure

Ventral corticospinal tract

Figure 18. Cervical cord (C2)—Weil, 18X

36

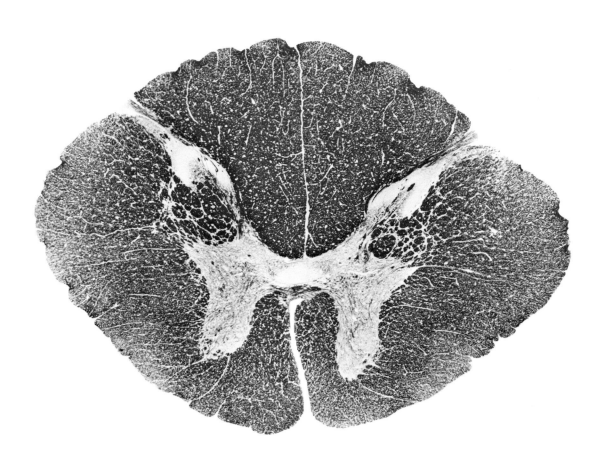

TRANSVERSE SECTIONS OF THE BRAIN STEM

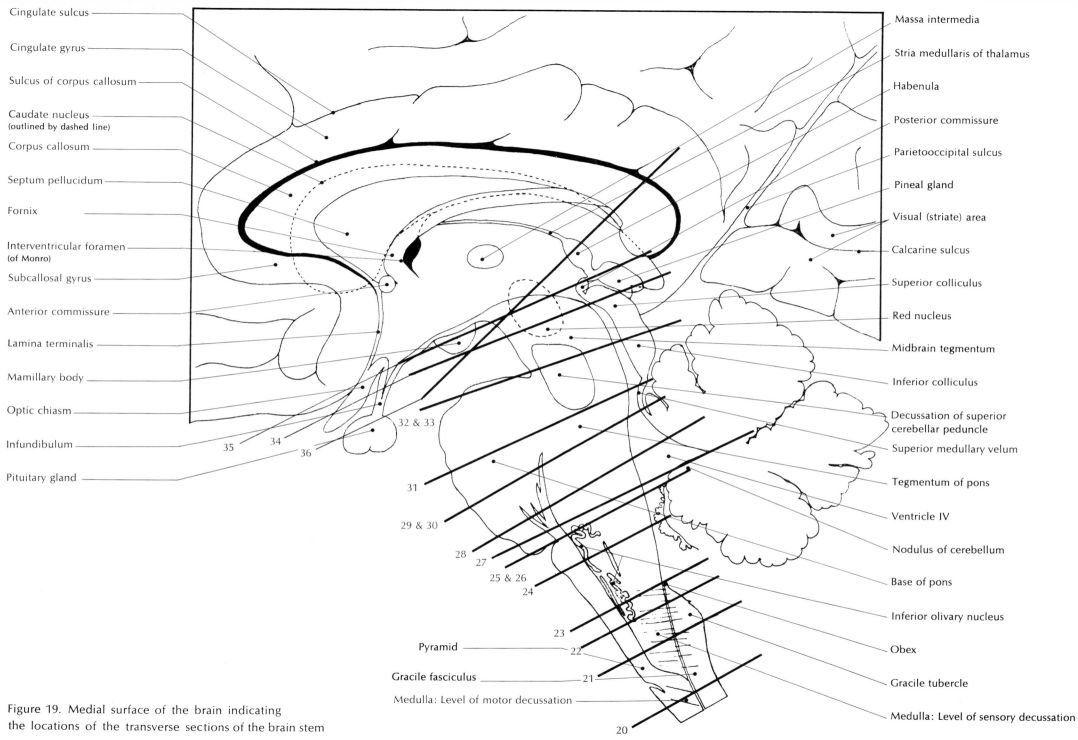

Cingulate sulcus

Cingulate gyrus

Sulcus of corpus callosum

Caudate nucleus
(outlined by dashed line)

Corpus callosum

Septum pellucidum

Fornix

Interventricular foramen
(of Monro)

Subcallosal gyrus

Anterior commissure

Lamina terminalis

Mamillary body

Optic chiasm

Infundibulum

Pituitary gland

Massa intermedia

Stria medullaris of thalamus

Habenula

Posterior commissure

Parietooccipital sulcus

Pineal gland

Visual (striate) area

Calcarine sulcus

Superior colliculus

Red nucleus

Midbrain tegmentum

Inferior colliculus

Decussation of superior
cerebellar peduncle

Superior medullary velum

Tegmentum of pons

Ventricle IV

Nodulus of cerebellum

Base of pons

Inferior olivary nucleus

Obex

Gracile tubercle

Medulla: Level of sensory decussation

Pyramid

Gracile fasciculus

Medulla: Level of motor decussation

35   34   36   32 & 33   31   29 & 30   28   27   25 & 26   24   23   22   21   20

Figure 19. Medial surface of the brain indicating
the locations of the transverse sections of the brain stem

39

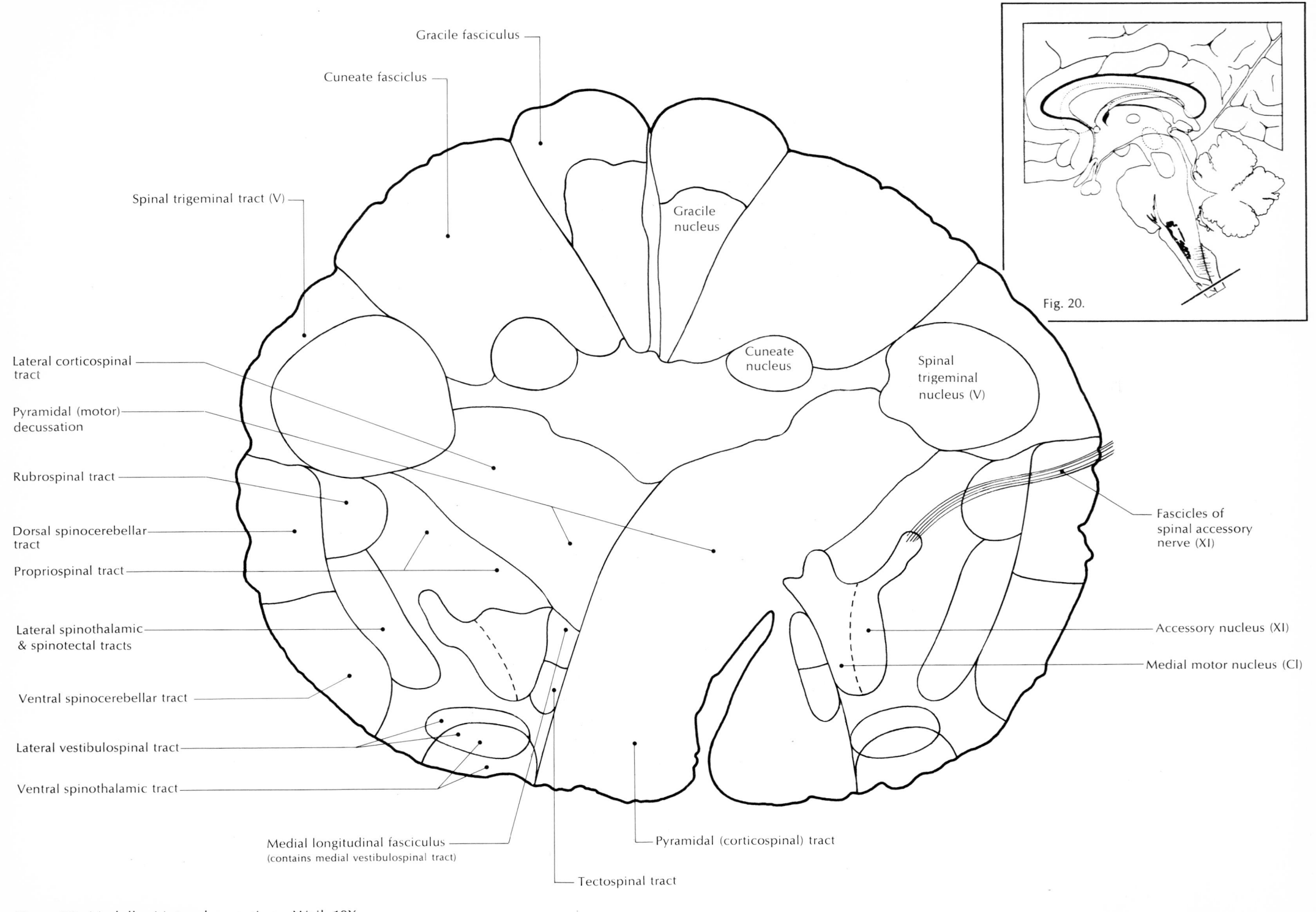

Gracile fasciculus

Cuneate fasciclus

Spinal trigeminal tract (V)

Gracile nucleus

Cuneate nucleus

Spinal trigeminal nucleus (V)

Lateral corticospinal tract

Pyramidal (motor) decussation

Rubrospinal tract

Dorsal spinocerebellar tract

Propriospinal tract

Lateral spinothalamic & spinotectal tracts

Ventral spinocerebellar tract

Lateral vestibulospinal tract

Ventral spinothalamic tract

Medial longitudinal fasciculus
(contains medial vestibulospinal tract)

Tectospinal tract

Pyramidal (corticospinal) tract

Fascicles of spinal accessory nerve (XI)

Accessory nucleus (XI)

Medial motor nucleus (CI)

Fig. 20.

Figure 20. Medulla: Motor decussation—Weil, 18X

40

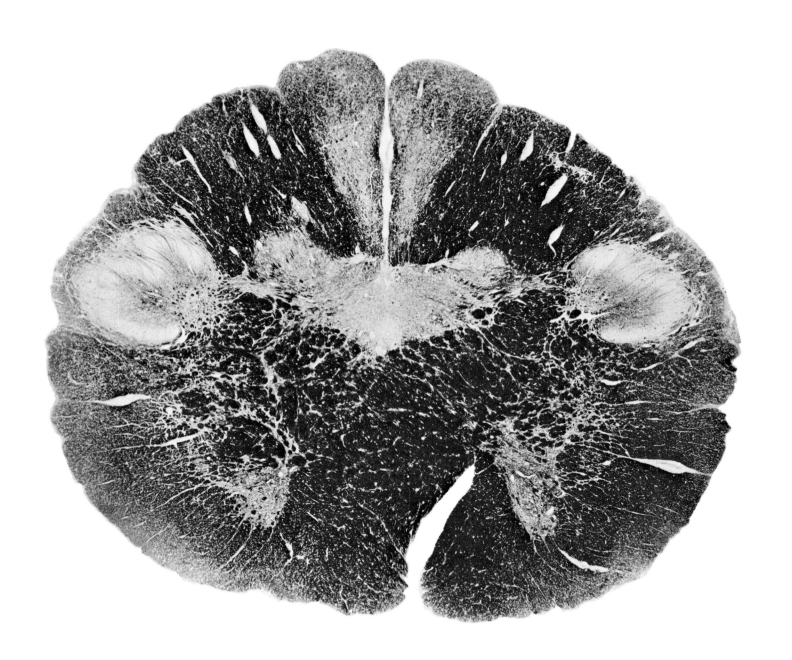

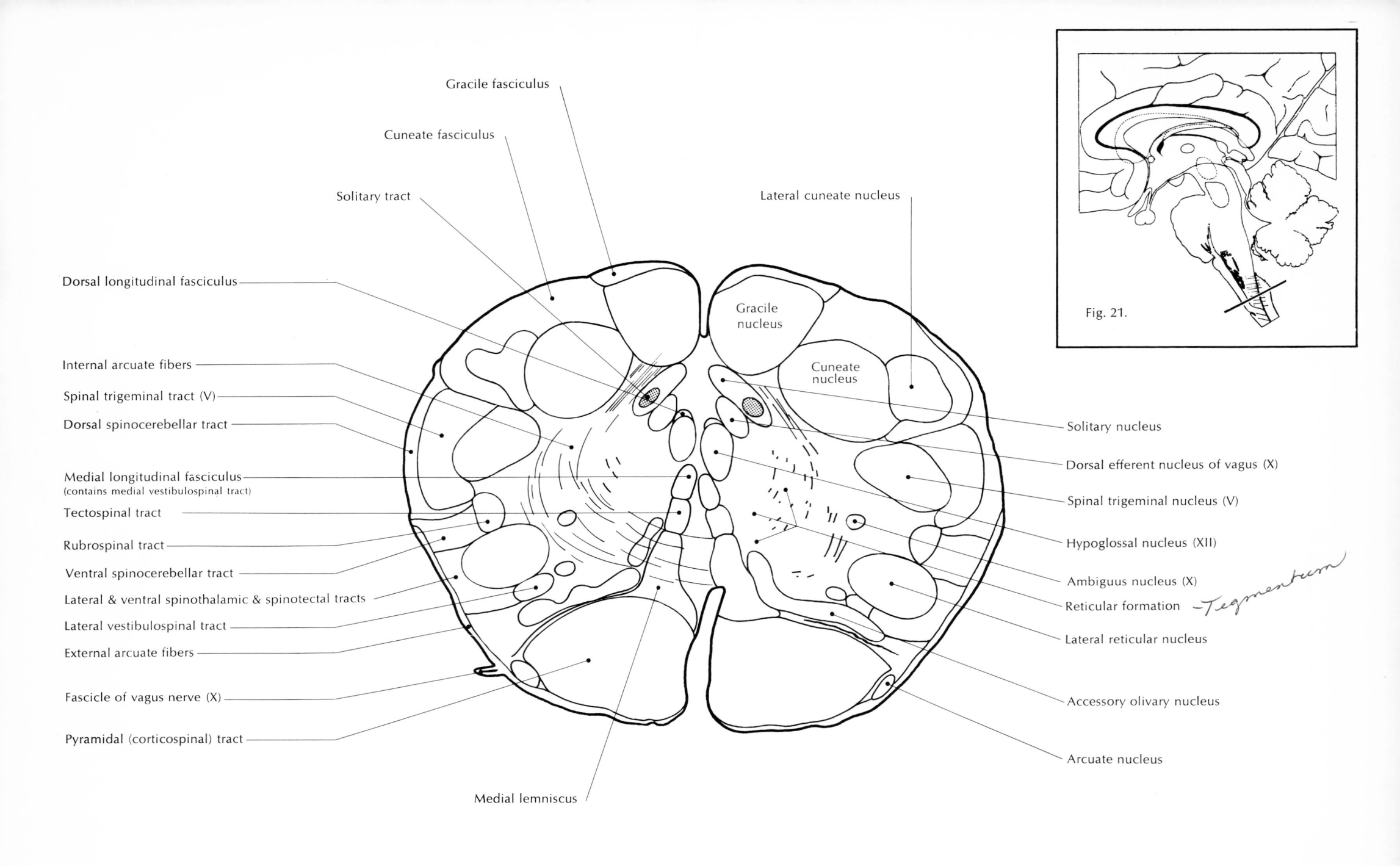

Gracile fasciculus

Cuneate fasciculus

Solitary tract

Lateral cuneate nucleus

Gracile nucleus

Cuneate nucleus

Dorsal longitudinal fasciculus

Internal arcuate fibers

Spinal trigeminal tract (V)

Dorsal spinocerebellar tract

Medial longitudinal fasciculus
(contains medial vestibulospinal tract)

Tectospinal tract

Rubrospinal tract

Ventral spinocerebellar tract

Lateral & ventral spinothalamic & spinotectal tracts

Lateral vestibulospinal tract

External arcuate fibers

Fascicle of vagus nerve (X)

Pyramidal (corticospinal) tract

Solitary nucleus

Dorsal efferent nucleus of vagus (X)

Spinal trigeminal nucleus (V)

Hypoglossal nucleus (XII)

Ambiguus nucleus (X)

Reticular formation   *Tegmentum*

Lateral reticular nucleus

Accessory olivary nucleus

Arcuate nucleus

Medial lemniscus

Fig. 21.

Figure 21. Medulla: Sensory decussation—Weil, 10X

42

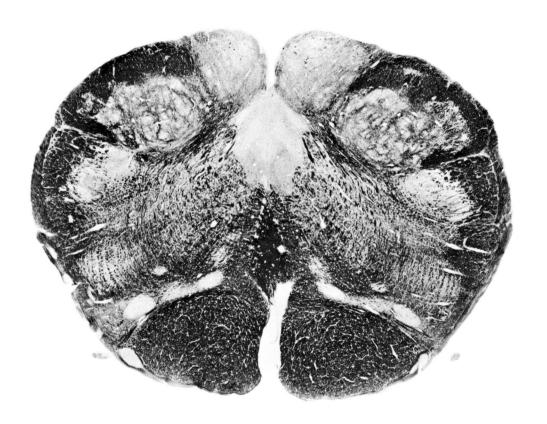

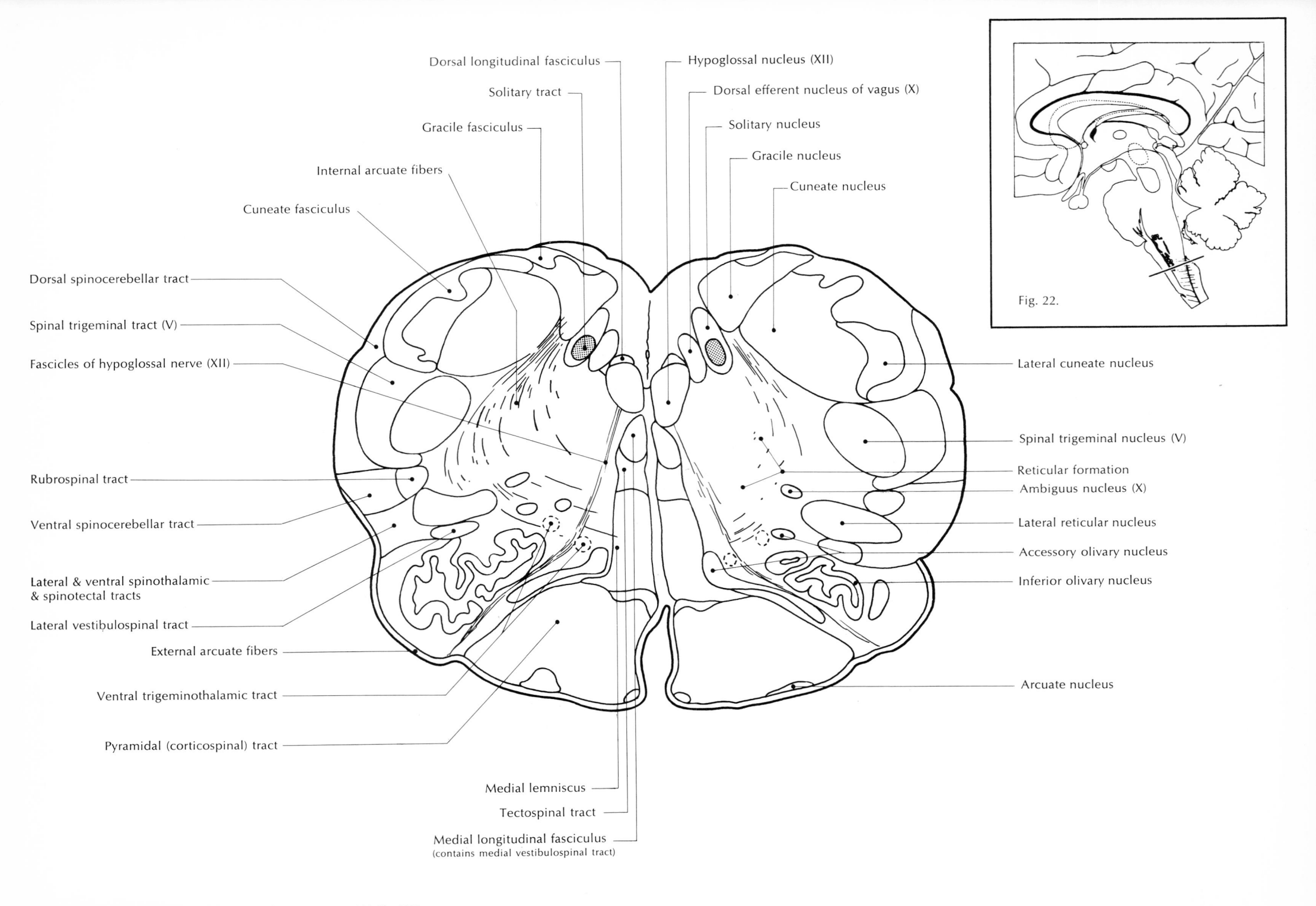

Dorsal longitudinal fasciculus

Solitary tract

Gracile fasciculus

Internal arcuate fibers

Cuneate fasciculus

Hypoglossal nucleus (XII)

Dorsal efferent nucleus of vagus (X)

Solitary nucleus

Gracile nucleus

Cuneate nucleus

Dorsal spinocerebellar tract

Spinal trigeminal tract (V)

Fascicles of hypoglossal nerve (XII)

Rubrospinal tract

Ventral spinocerebellar tract

Lateral & ventral spinothalamic & spinotectal tracts

Lateral vestibulospinal tract

External arcuate fibers

Ventral trigeminothalamic tract

Pyramidal (corticospinal) tract

Lateral cuneate nucleus

Spinal trigeminal nucleus (V)

Reticular formation

Ambiguus nucleus (X)

Lateral reticular nucleus

Accessory olivary nucleus

Inferior olivary nucleus

Arcuate nucleus

Medial lemniscus

Tectospinal tract

Medial longitudinal fasciculus
(contains medial vestibulospinal tract)

Fig. 22.

Figure 22. Medulla: Rostral sensory decussation—Weil, 10X

44

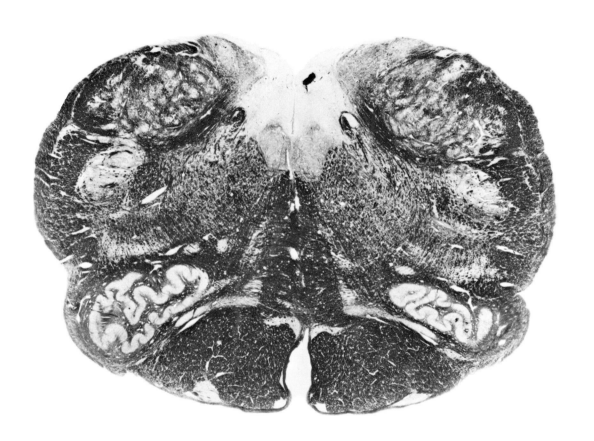

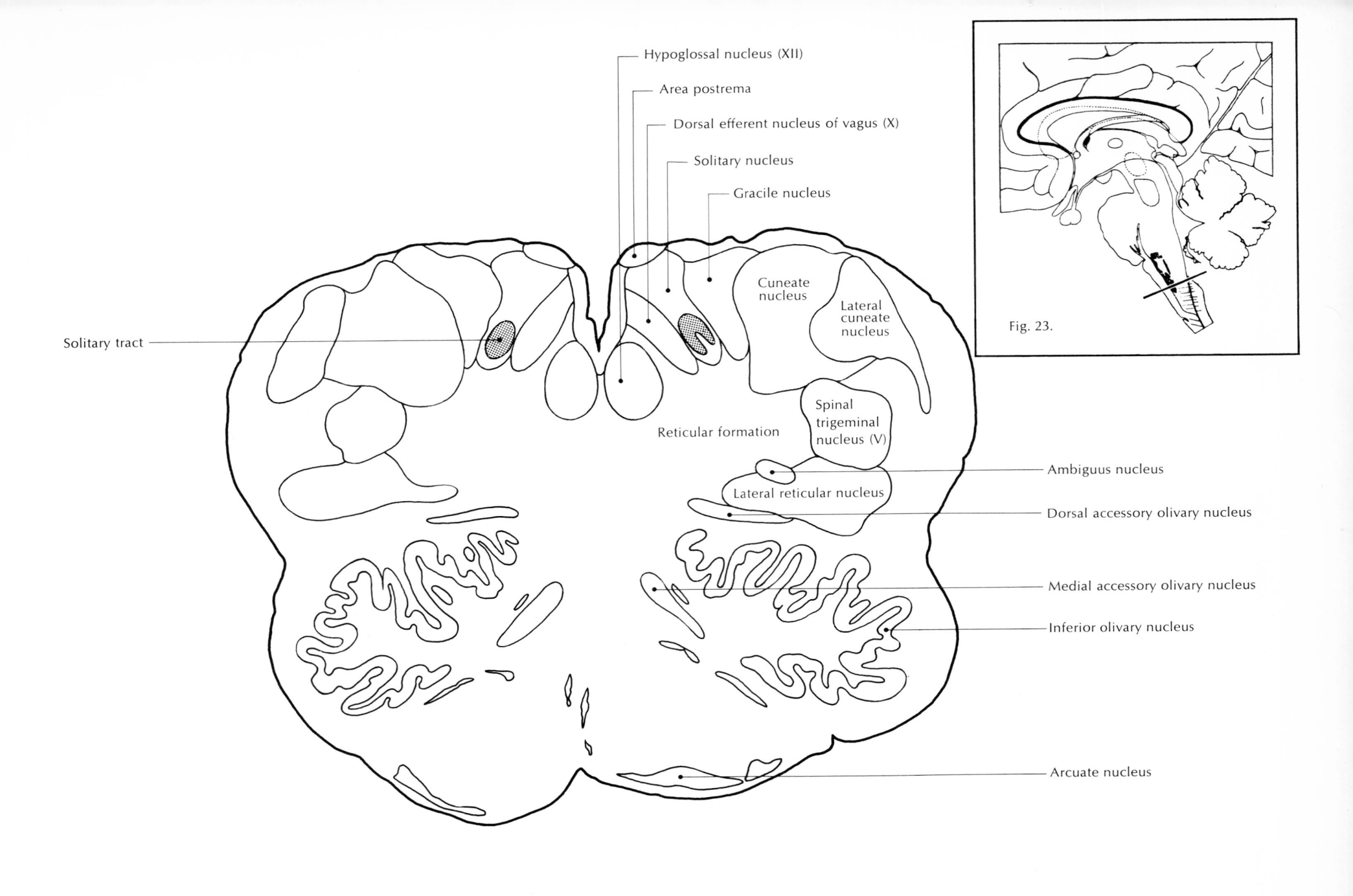

Hypoglossal nucleus (XII)

Area postrema

Dorsal efferent nucleus of vagus (X)

Solitary nucleus

Gracile nucleus

Cuneate nucleus

Lateral cuneate nucleus

Solitary tract

Spinal trigeminal nucleus (V)

Reticular formation

Ambiguus nucleus

Lateral reticular nucleus

Dorsal accessory olivary nucleus

Medial accessory olivary nucleus

Inferior olivary nucleus

Arcuate nucleus

Fig. 23.

Figure 23. Medulla (obex; transition from closed to open medulla): Level of cranial nerve nuclei X and XII—Nissl, 10X

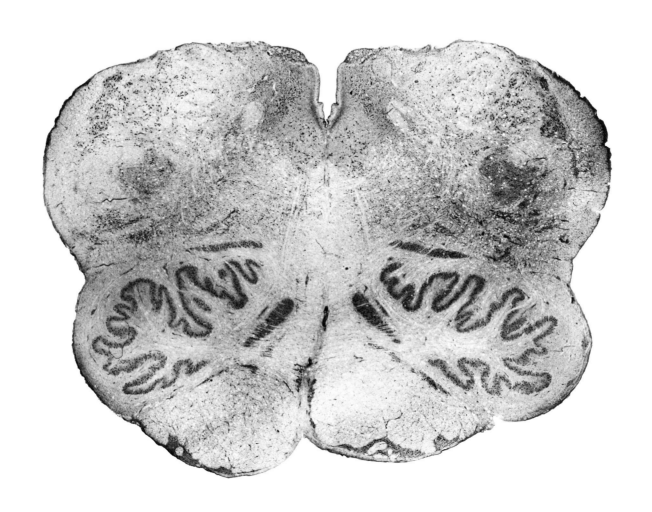

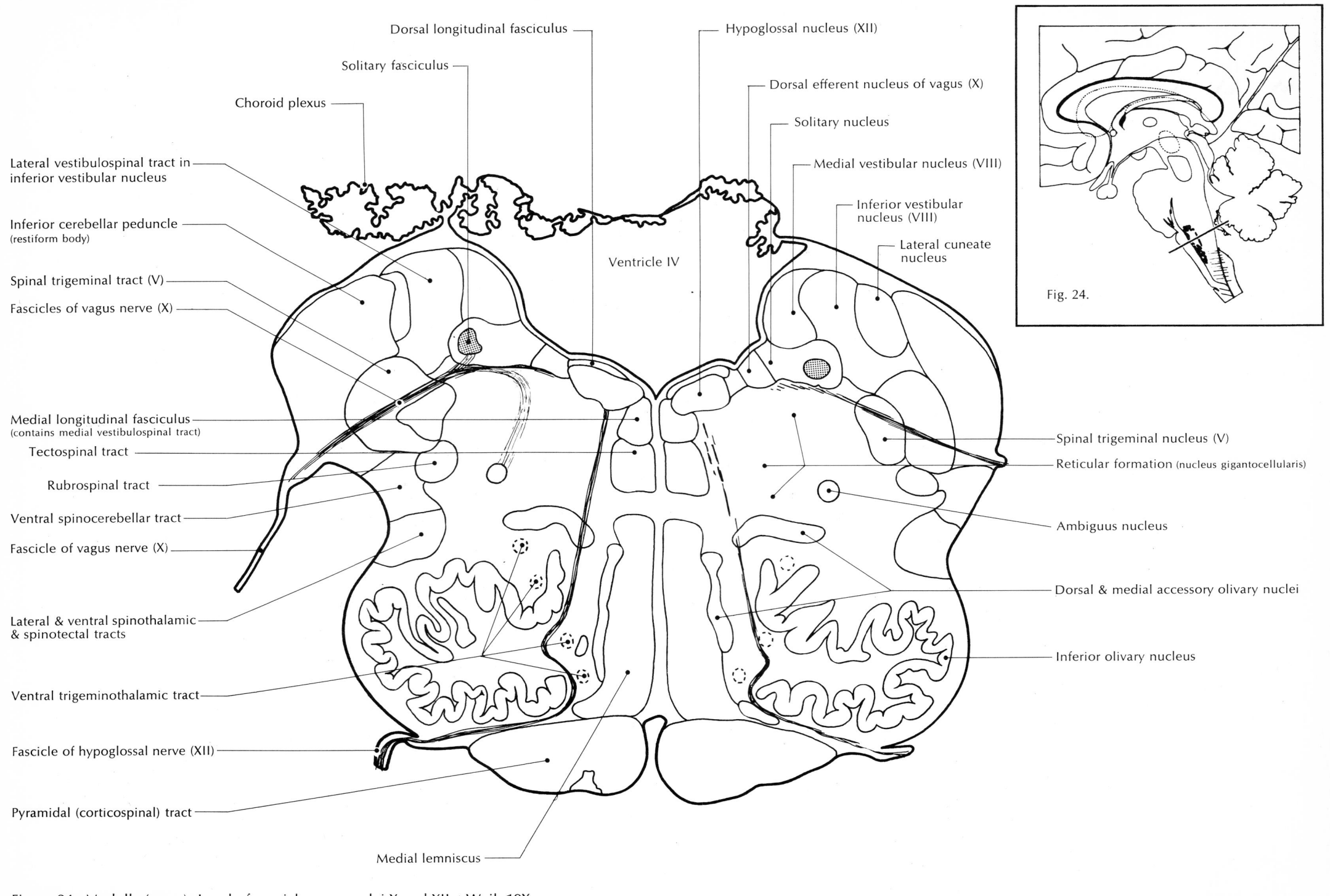

Dorsal longitudinal fasciculus

Solitary fasciculus

Choroid plexus

Hypoglossal nucleus (XII)

Dorsal efferent nucleus of vagus (X)

Solitary nucleus

Medial vestibular nucleus (VIII)

Inferior vestibular nucleus (VIII)

Lateral cuneate nucleus

Lateral vestibulospinal tract in inferior vestibular nucleus

Inferior cerebellar peduncle (restiform body)

Spinal trigeminal tract (V)

Fascicles of vagus nerve (X)

Ventricle IV

Medial longitudinal fasciculus (contains medial vestibulospinal tract)

Tectospinal tract

Rubrospinal tract

Ventral spinocerebellar tract

Fascicle of vagus nerve (X)

Lateral & ventral spinothalamic & spinotectal tracts

Ventral trigeminothalamic tract

Fascicle of hypoglossal nerve (XII)

Pyramidal (corticospinal) tract

Medial lemniscus

Spinal trigeminal nucleus (V)

Reticular formation (nucleus gigantocellularis)

Ambiguus nucleus

Dorsal & medial accessory olivary nuclei

Inferior olivary nucleus

Fig. 24.

Figure 24. Medulla (open): Level of cranial nerve nuclei X and XII—Weil, 10X

48

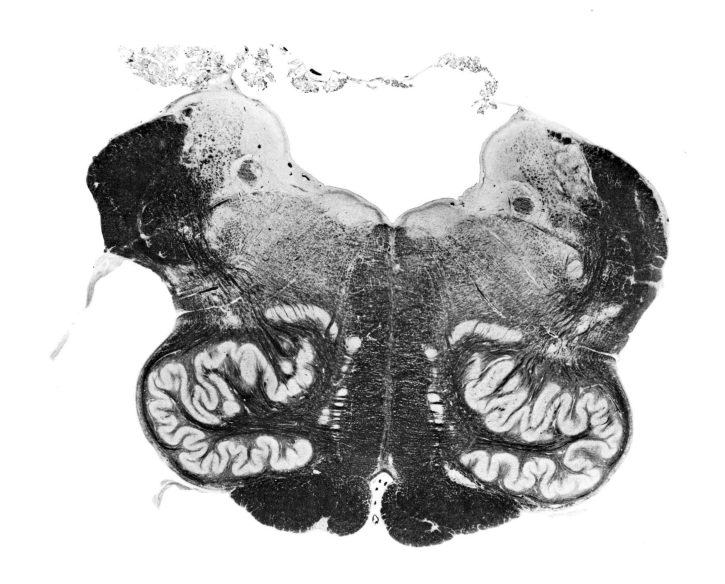

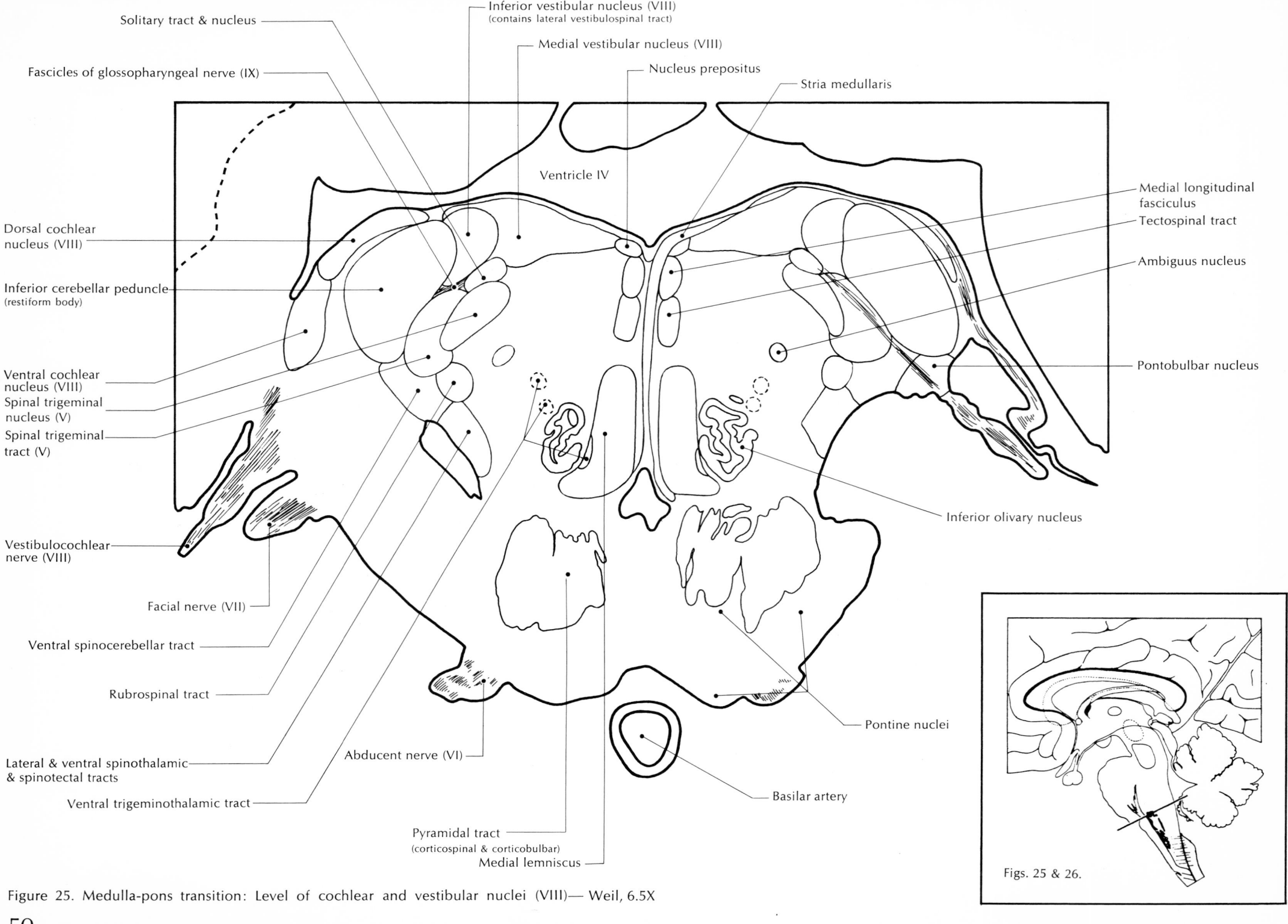

Solitary tract & nucleus

Fascicles of glossopharyngeal nerve (IX)

Dorsal cochlear nucleus (VIII)

Inferior cerebellar peduncle (restiform body)

Ventral cochlear nucleus (VIII)

Spinal trigeminal nucleus (V)

Spinal trigeminal tract (V)

Vestibulocochlear nerve (VIII)

Facial nerve (VII)

Ventral spinocerebellar tract

Rubrospinal tract

Lateral & ventral spinothalamic & spinotectal tracts

Ventral trigeminothalamic tract

Abducent nerve (VI)

Pyramidal tract (corticospinal & corticobulbar)

Medial lemniscus

Inferior vestibular nucleus (VIII) (contains lateral vestibulospinal tract)

Medial vestibular nucleus (VIII)

Nucleus prepositus

Stria medullaris

Ventricle IV

Medial longitudinal fasciculus

Tectospinal tract

Ambiguus nucleus

Pontobulbar nucleus

Inferior olivary nucleus

Pontine nuclei

Basilar artery

Figs. 25 & 26.

Figure 25. Medulla-pons transition: Level of cochlear and vestibular nuclei (VIII)— Weil, 6.5X

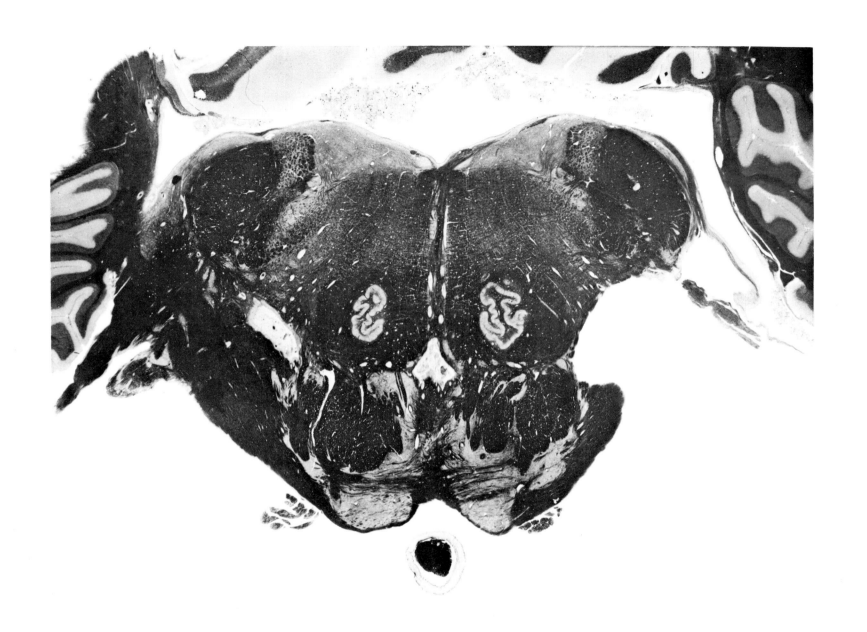

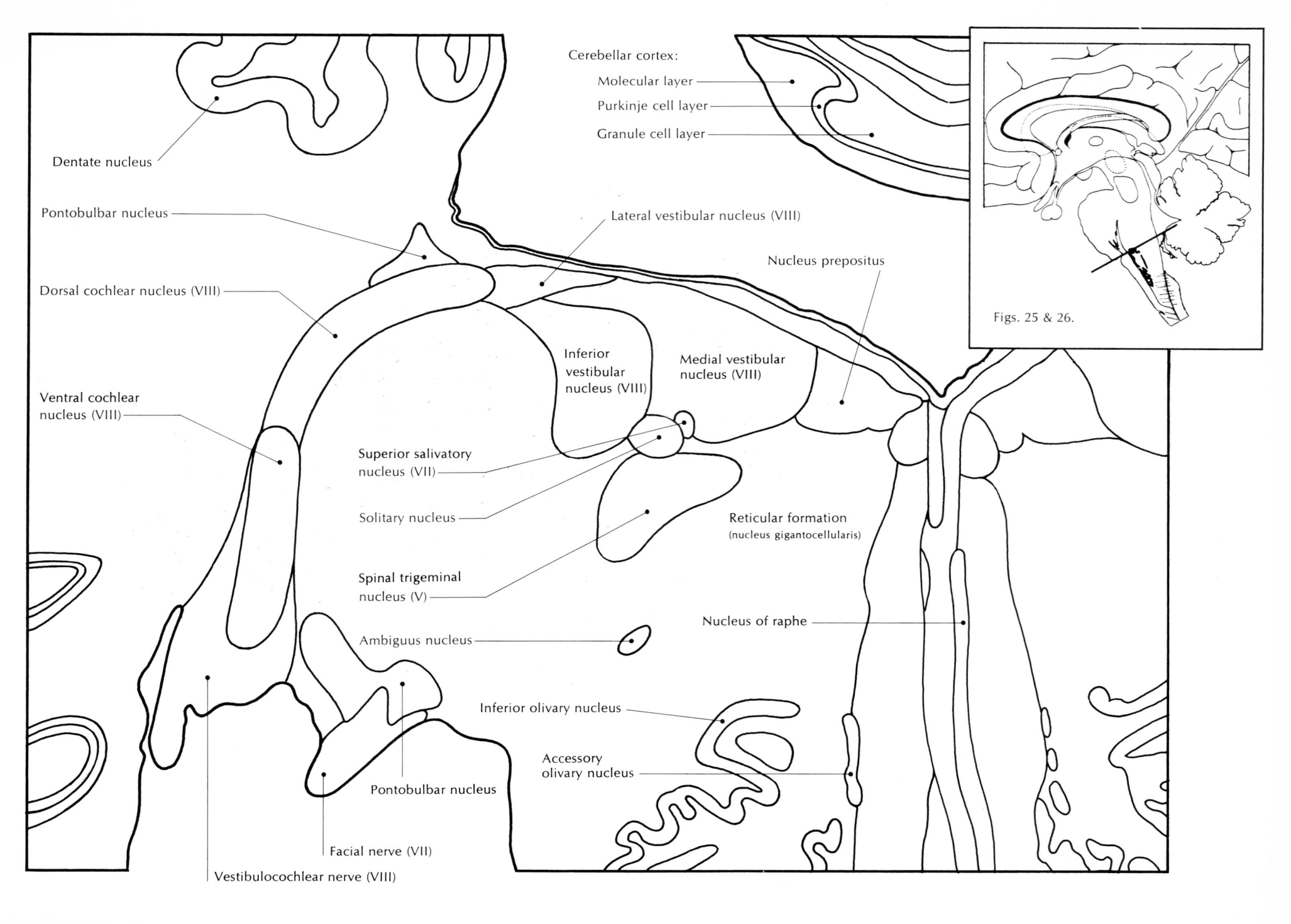

Cerebellar cortex:

Molecular layer

Purkinje cell layer

Granule cell layer

Dentate nucleus

Pontobulbar nucleus

Lateral vestibular nucleus (VIII)

Nucleus prepositus

Dorsal cochlear nucleus (VIII)

Inferior vestibular nucleus (VIII)

Medial vestibular nucleus (VIII)

Figs. 25 & 26.

Ventral cochlear nucleus (VIII)

Superior salivatory nucleus (VII)

Solitary nucleus

Reticular formation (nucleus gigantocellularis)

Spinal trigeminal nucleus (V)

Nucleus of raphe

Ambiguus nucleus

Inferior olivary nucleus

Accessory olivary nucleus

Pontobulbar nucleus

Facial nerve (VII)

Vestibulocochlear nerve (VIII)

Figure 26. Medulla-pons transition: Level of cochlear and vestibular nuclei (VIII)—Nissl, 14X

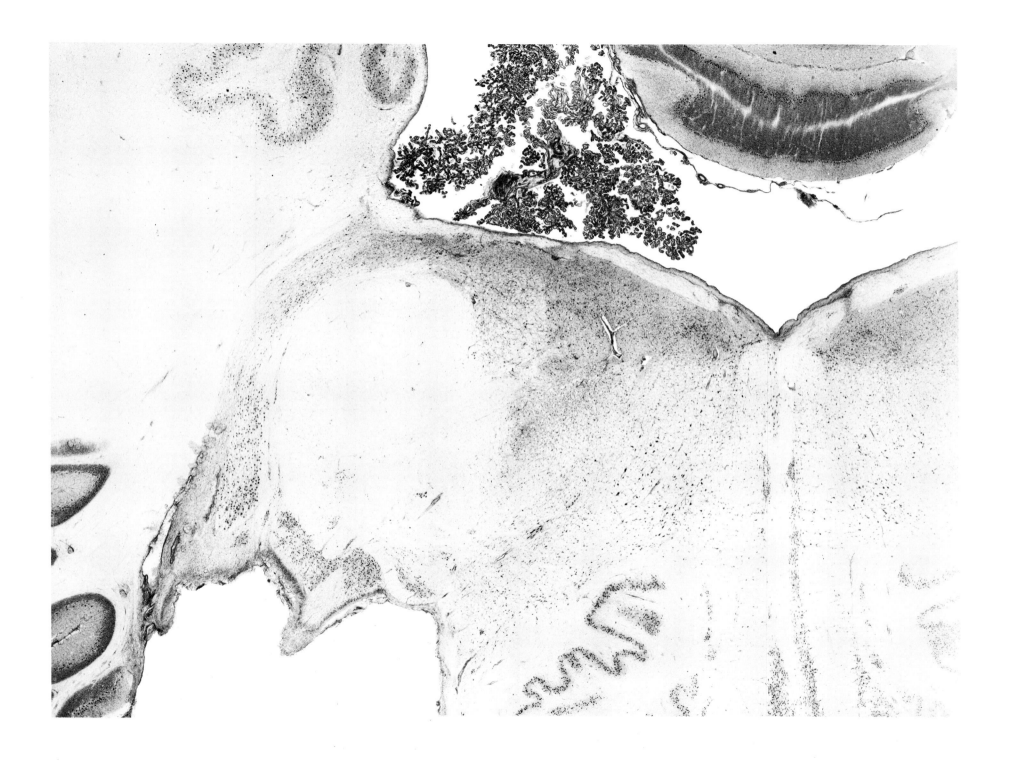

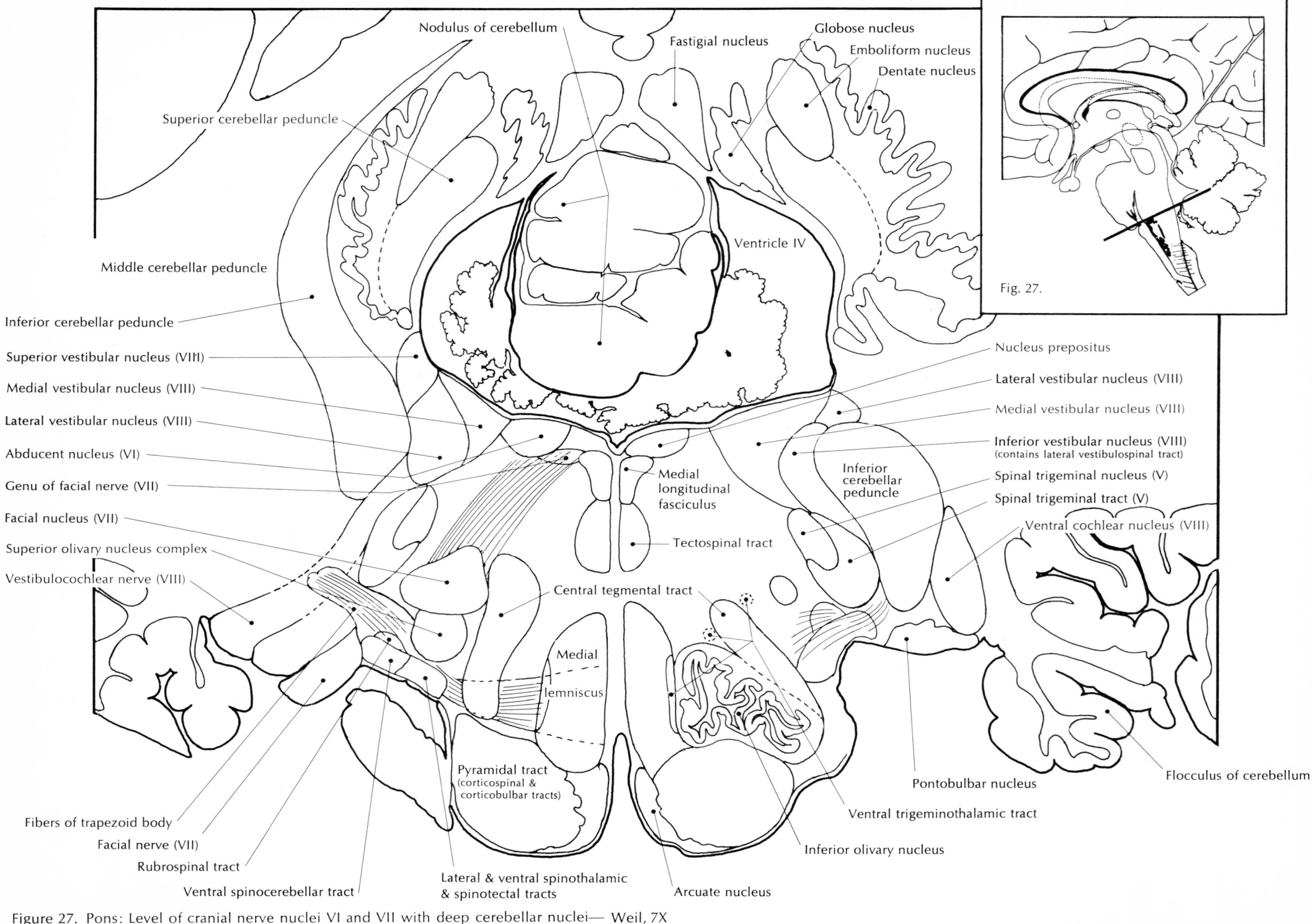

Nodulus of cerebellum

Fastigial nucleus

Globose nucleus

Emboliform nucleus

Dentate nucleus

Superior cerebellar peduncle

Middle cerebellar peduncle

Ventricle IV

Inferior cerebellar peduncle

Nucleus prepositus

Superior vestibular nucleus (VIII)

Lateral vestibular nucleus (VIII)

Medial vestibular nucleus (VIII)

Medial vestibular nucleus (VIII)

Lateral vestibular nucleus (VIII)

Inferior vestibular nucleus (VIII)
(contains lateral vestibulospinal tract)

Abducent nucleus (VI)

Inferior cerebellar peduncle

Genu of facial nerve (VII)

Medial longitudinal fasciculus

Spinal trigeminal nucleus (V)

Facial nucleus (VII)

Spinal trigeminal tract (V)

Superior olivary nucleus complex

Ventral cochlear nucleus (VIII)

Vestibulocochlear nerve (VIII)

Tectospinal tract

Central tegmental tract

Medial lemniscus

Pyramidal tract
(corticospinal & corticobulbar tracts)

Flocculus of cerebellum

Pontobulbar nucleus

Fibers of trapezoid body

Ventral trigeminothalamic tract

Facial nerve (VII)

Inferior olivary nucleus

Rubrospinal tract

Ventral spinocerebellar tract

Lateral & ventral spinothalamic & spinotectal tracts

Arcuate nucleus

Fig. 27.

Figure 27. Pons: Level of cranial nerve nuclei VI and VII with deep cerebellar nuclei— Weil, 7X

54

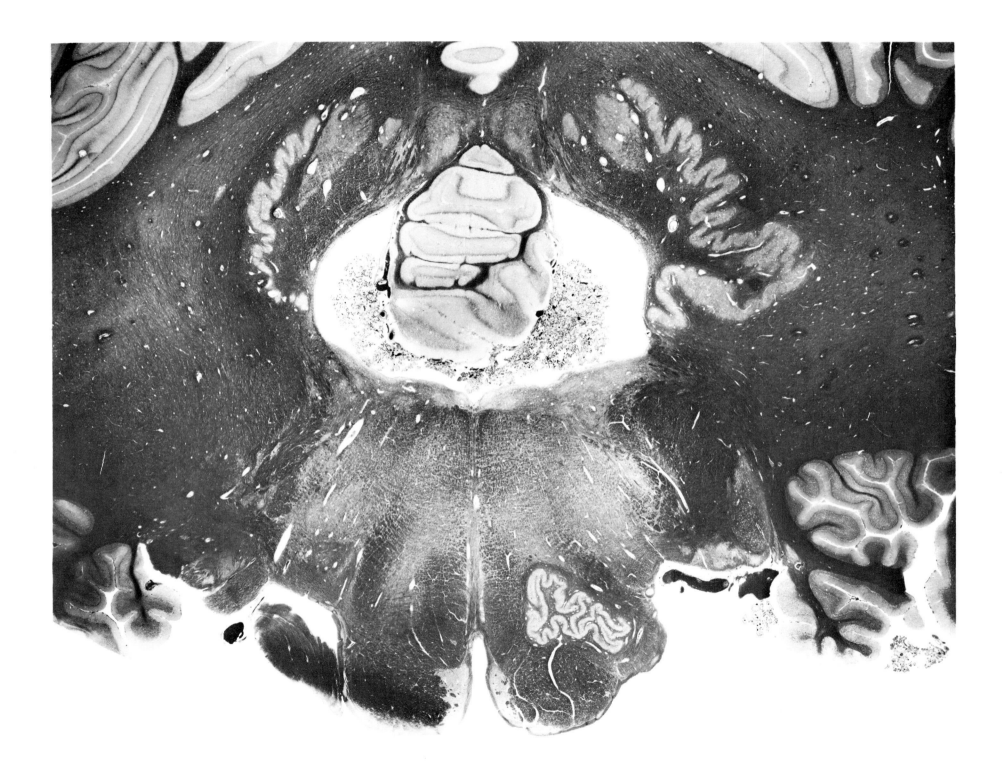

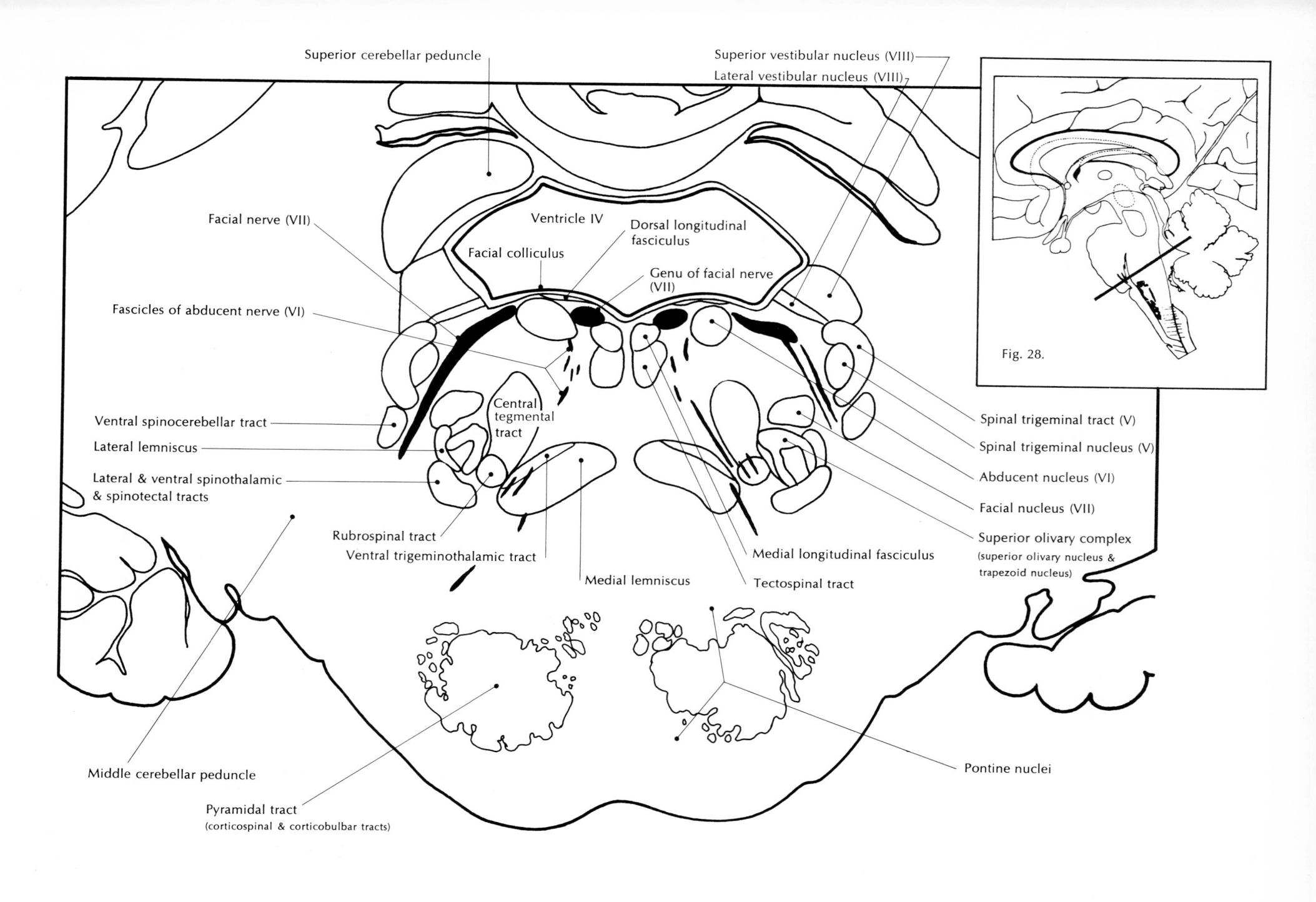

Superior cerebellar peduncle

Superior vestibular nucleus (VIII)

Lateral vestibular nucleus (VIII)

Facial nerve (VII)

Ventricle IV

Dorsal longitudinal fasciculus

Facial colliculus

Genu of facial nerve (VII)

Fascicles of abducent nerve (VI)

Central tegmental tract

Ventral spinocerebellar tract

Spinal trigeminal tract (V)

Lateral lemniscus

Spinal trigeminal nucleus (V)

Lateral & ventral spinothalamic & spinotectal tracts

Abducent nucleus (VI)

Rubrospinal tract

Facial nucleus (VII)

Ventral trigeminothalamic tract

Medial longitudinal fasciculus

Superior olivary complex (superior olivary nucleus & trapezoid nucleus)

Medial lemniscus

Tectospinal tract

Fig. 28.

Middle cerebellar peduncle

Pontine nuclei

Pyramidal tract (corticospinal & corticobulbar tracts)

Figure 28. Pons: Level of cranial nerve nuclei VI and VII—Weil, 6.5X

56

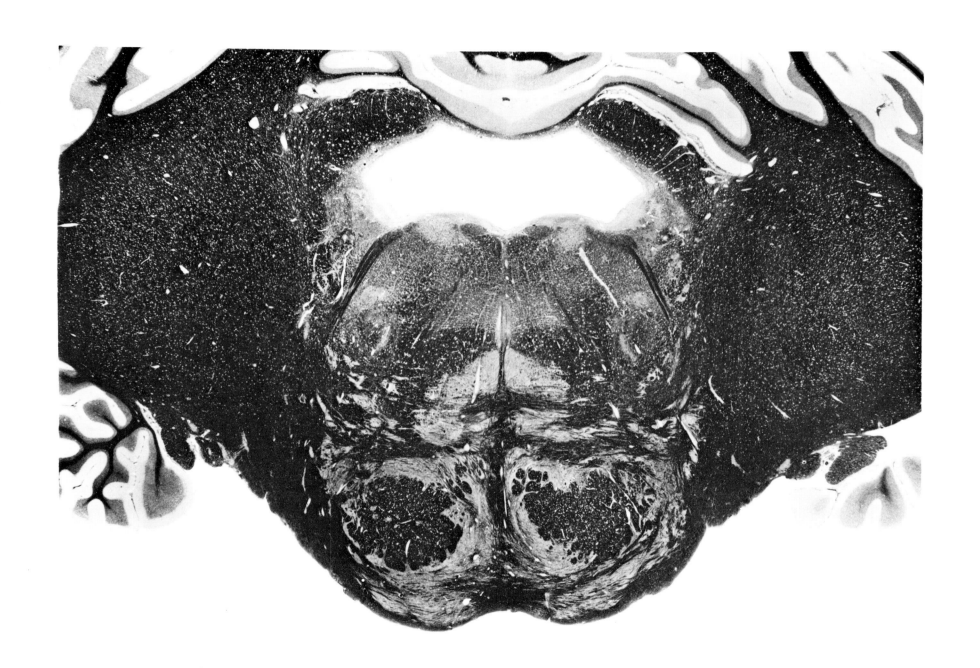

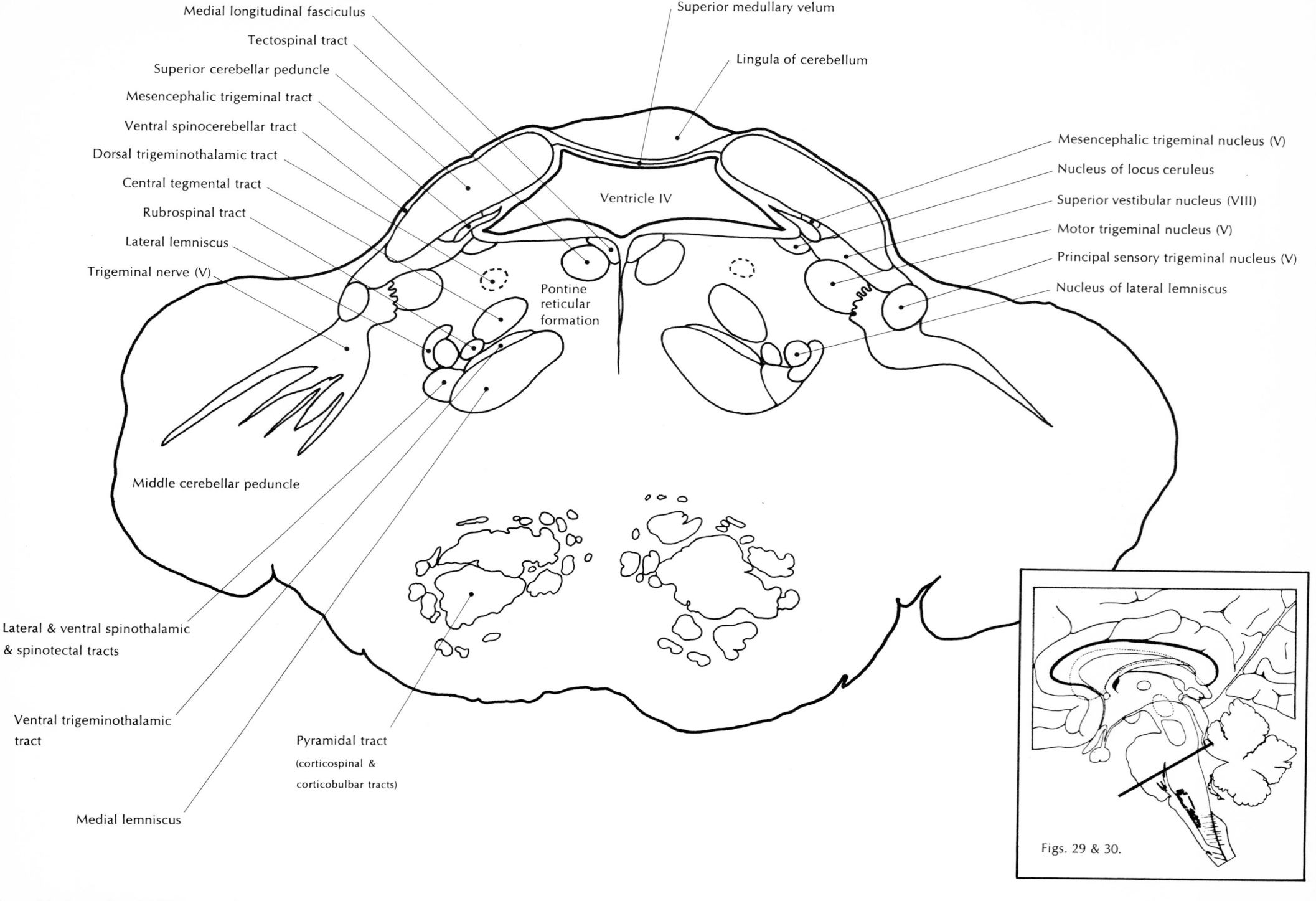

Medial longitudinal fasciculus

Tectospinal tract

Superior cerebellar peduncle

Mesencephalic trigeminal tract

Ventral spinocerebellar tract

Dorsal trigeminothalamic tract

Central tegmental tract

Rubrospinal tract

Lateral lemniscus

Trigeminal nerve (V)

Superior medullary velum

Lingula of cerebellum

Ventricle IV

Pontine reticular formation

Mesencephalic trigeminal nucleus (V)

Nucleus of locus ceruleus

Superior vestibular nucleus (VIII)

Motor trigeminal nucleus (V)

Principal sensory trigeminal nucleus (V)

Nucleus of lateral lemniscus

Middle cerebellar peduncle

Lateral & ventral spinothalamic & spinotectal tracts

Ventral trigeminothalamic tract

Pyramidal tract (corticospinal & corticobulbar tracts)

Medial lemniscus

Figs. 29 & 30.

Figure 29. Pons: Level of motor and principal sensory nuclei of cranial nerve V—Weil, 6.5X

58

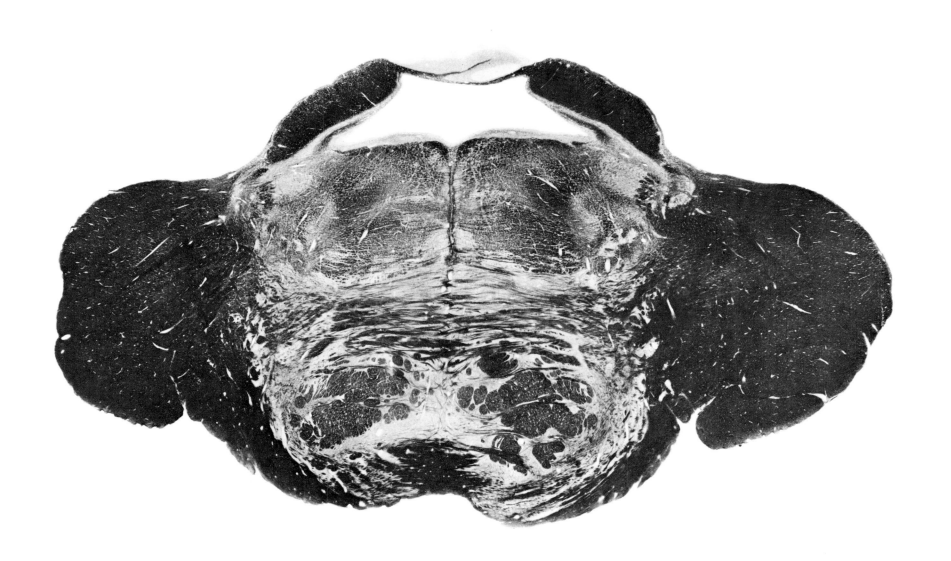

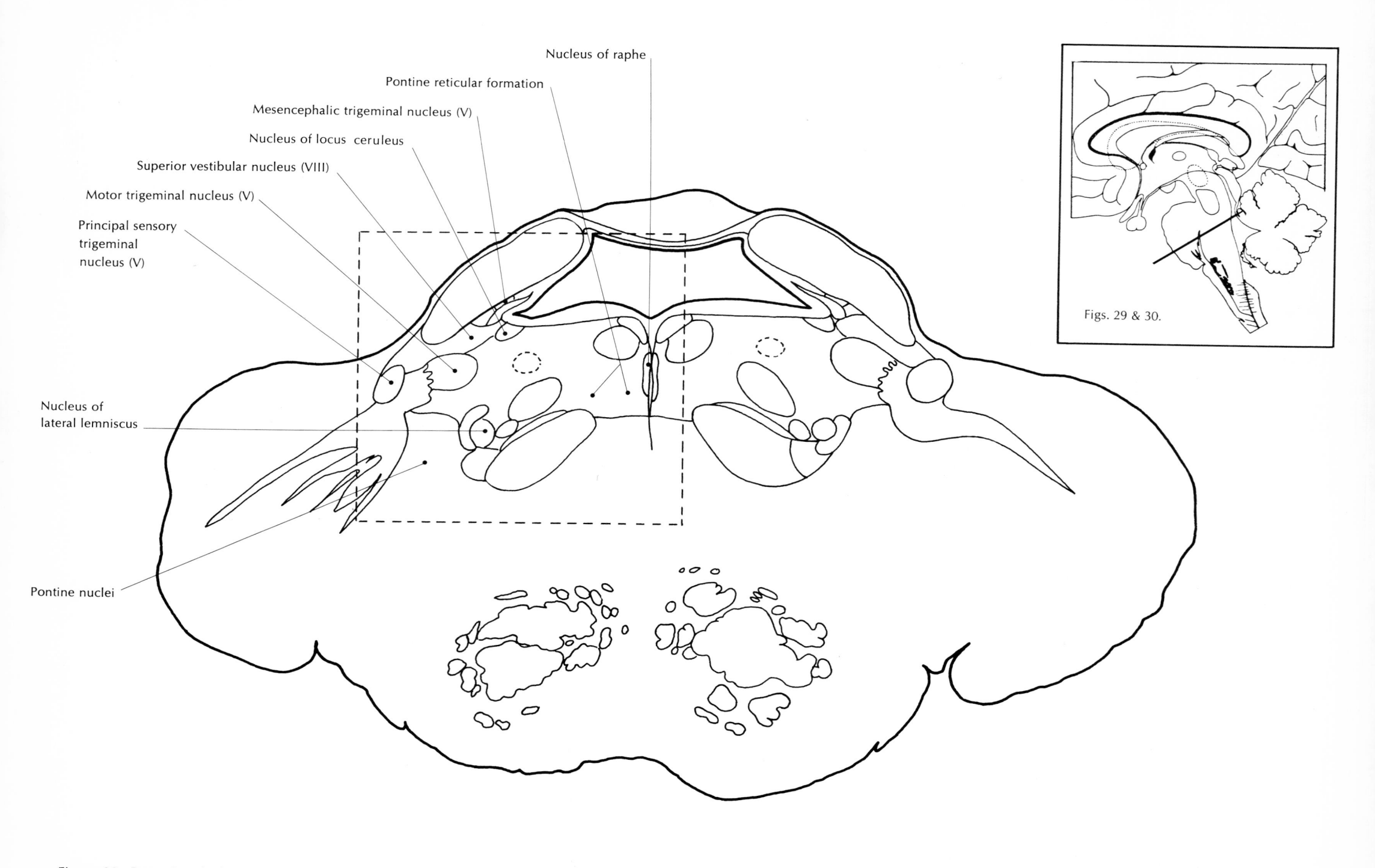

Nucleus of raphe

Pontine reticular formation

Mesencephalic trigeminal nucleus (V)

Nucleus of locus ceruleus

Superior vestibular nucleus (VIII)

Motor trigeminal nucleus (V)

Principal sensory trigeminal nucleus (V)

Nucleus of lateral lemniscus

Pontine nuclei

Figs. 29 & 30.

Figure 30. Pons: Level of motor and principal sensory nuclei of cranial nerve V—Nissl, 20X

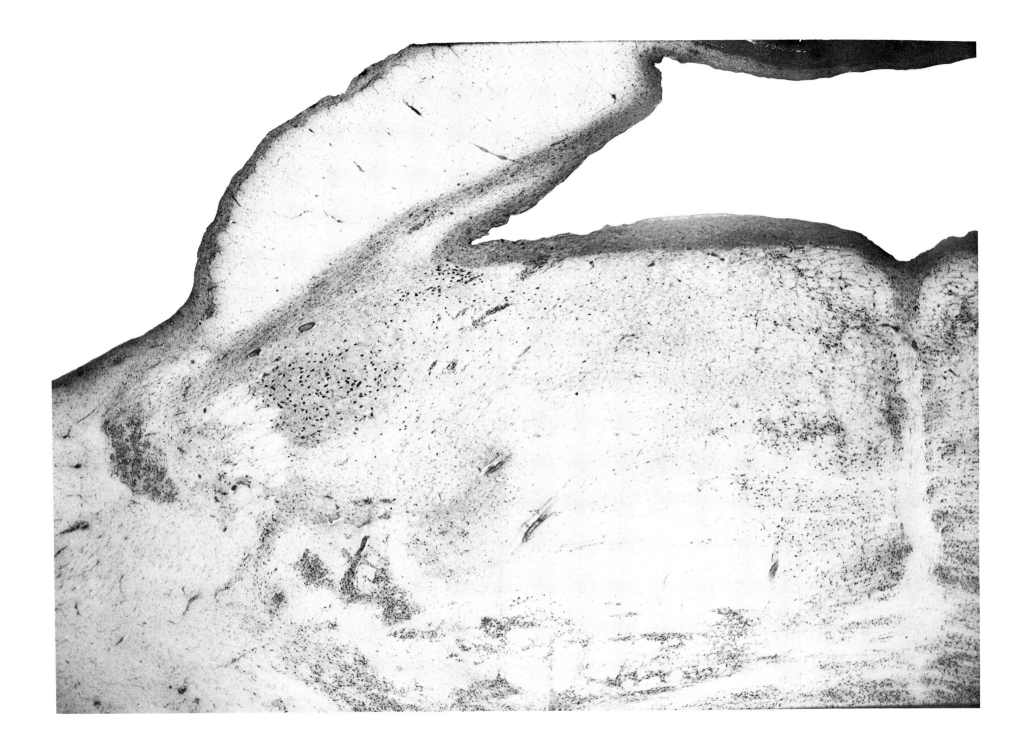

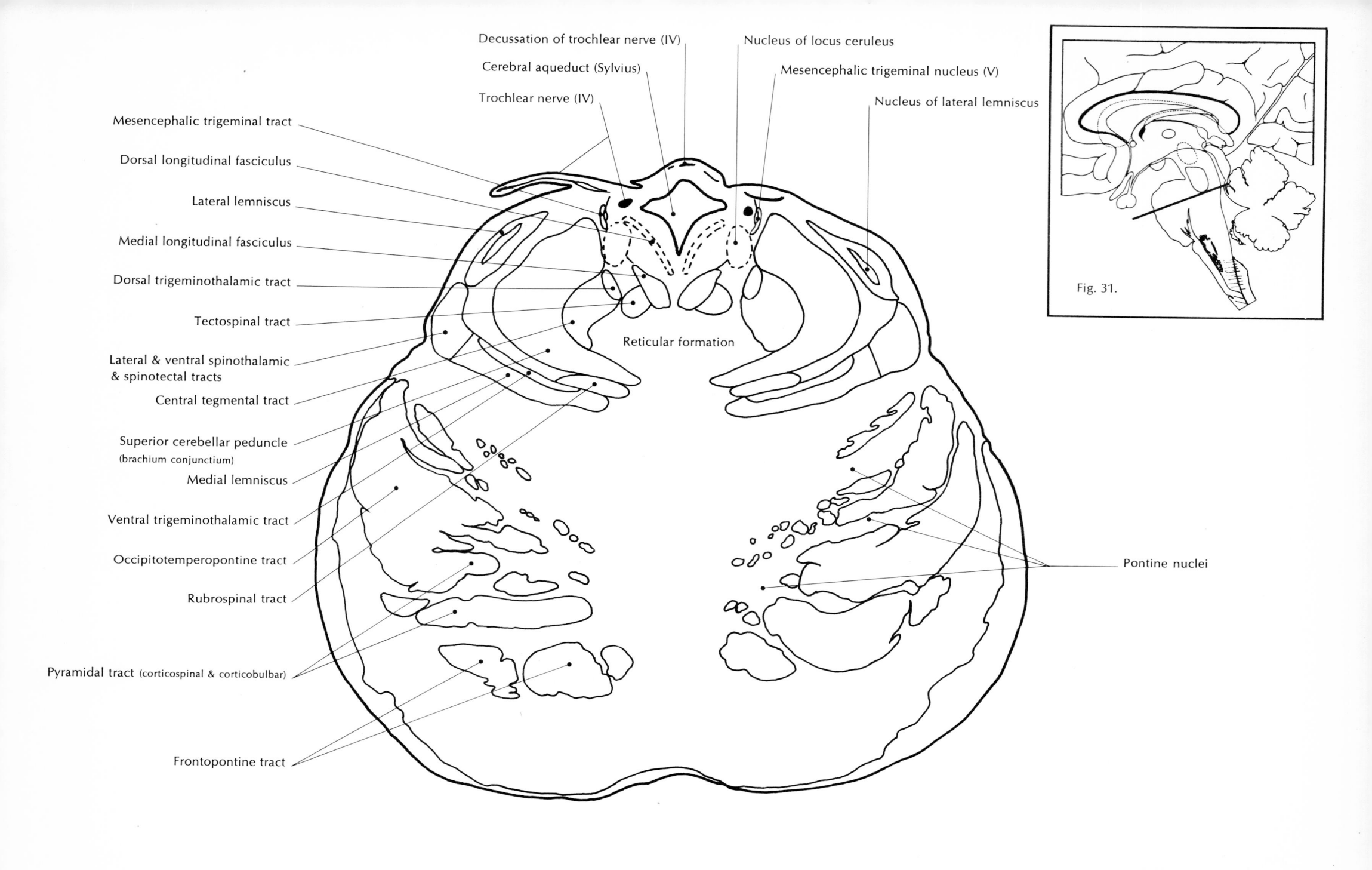

Decussation of trochlear nerve (IV)

Cerebral aqueduct (Sylvius)

Trochlear nerve (IV)

Nucleus of locus ceruleus

Mesencephalic trigeminal nucleus (V)

Nucleus of lateral lemniscus

Mesencephalic trigeminal tract

Dorsal longitudinal fasciculus

Lateral lemniscus

Medial longitudinal fasciculus

Dorsal trigeminothalamic tract

Tectospinal tract

Lateral & ventral spinothalamic
& spinotectal tracts

Central tegmental tract

Superior cerebellar peduncle
(brachium conjunctium)

Medial lemniscus

Ventral trigeminothalamic tract

Occipitotemperopontine tract

Rubrospinal tract

Pyramidal tract (corticospinal & corticobulbar)

Frontopontine tract

Reticular formation

Pontine nuclei

Fig. 31.

Figure 31. Pons: Isthmus, contains medial longitudinal fasciculus interconnecting the extraocular muscle motor nuclei, III, IV, and VI—Weil, 6.5X

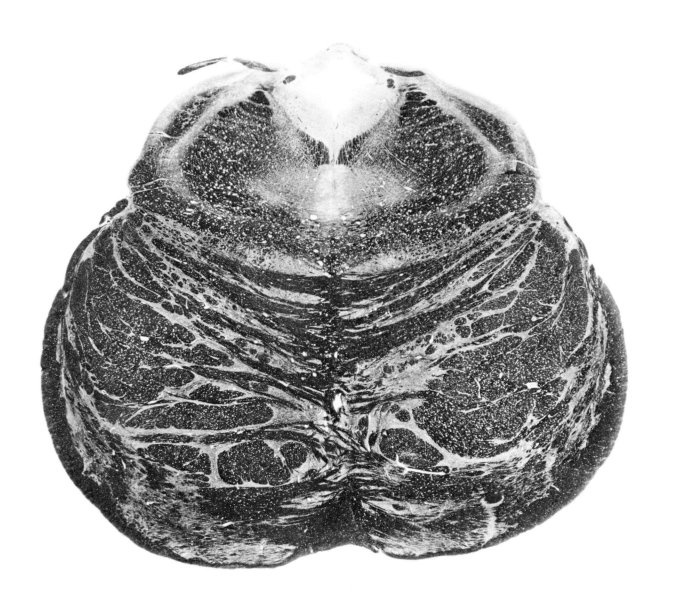

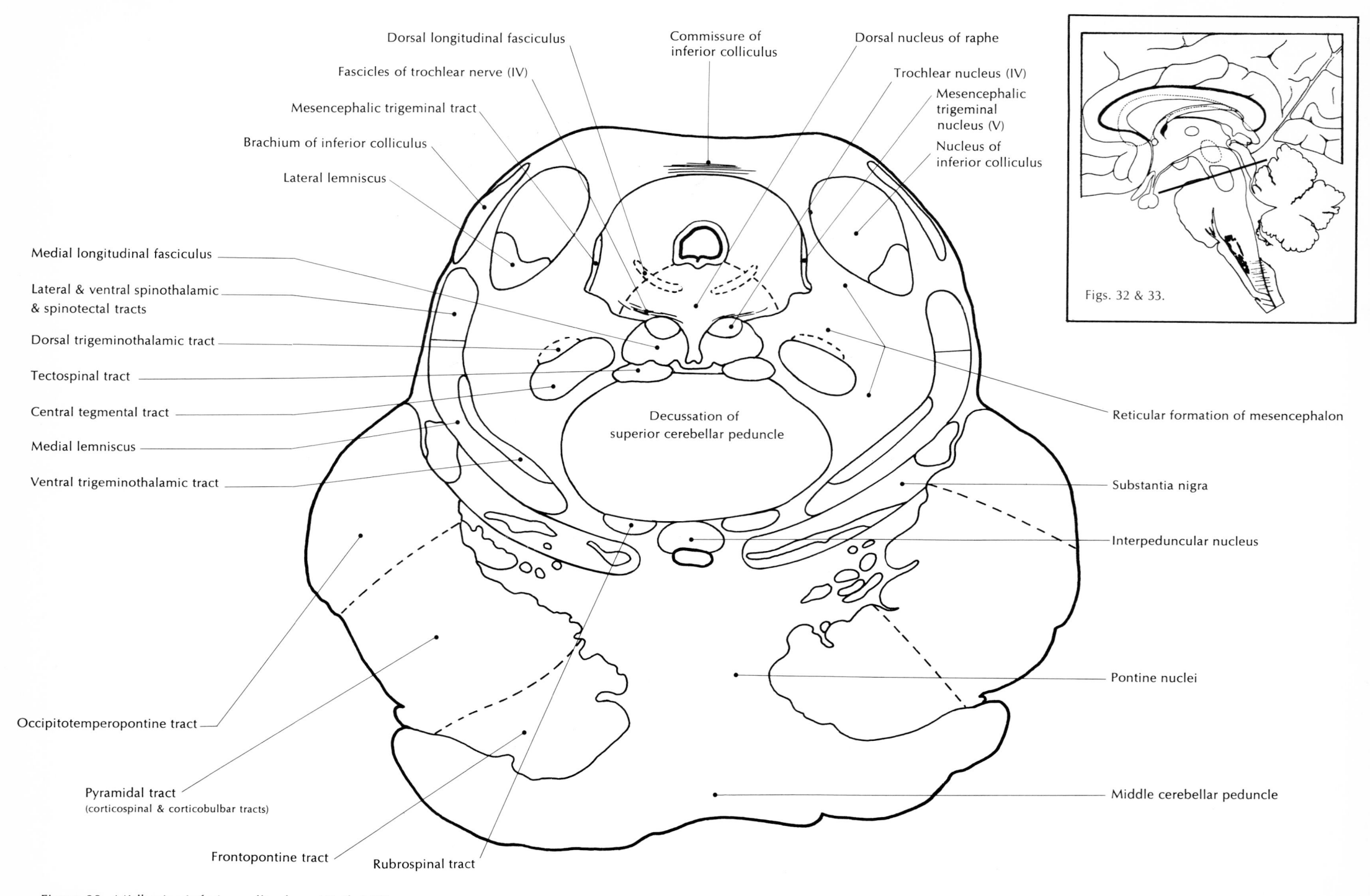

Dorsal longitudinal fasciculus

Fascicles of trochlear nerve (IV)

Mesencephalic trigeminal tract

Brachium of inferior colliculus

Lateral lemniscus

Commissure of inferior colliculus

Dorsal nucleus of raphe

Trochlear nucleus (IV)

Mesencephalic trigeminal nucleus (V)

Nucleus of inferior colliculus

Medial longitudinal fasciculus

Lateral & ventral spinothalamic & spinotectal tracts

Dorsal trigeminothalamic tract

Tectospinal tract

Central tegmental tract

Medial lemniscus

Ventral trigeminothalamic tract

Decussation of superior cerebellar peduncle

Reticular formation of mesencephalon

Substantia nigra

Interpeduncular nucleus

Pontine nuclei

Middle cerebellar peduncle

Occipitotemperopontine tract

Pyramidal tract
(corticospinal & corticobulbar tracts)

Frontopontine tract

Rubrospinal tract

Figs. 32 & 33.

Figure 32. Midbrain: Inferior colliculus—Weil, 6.5X

64

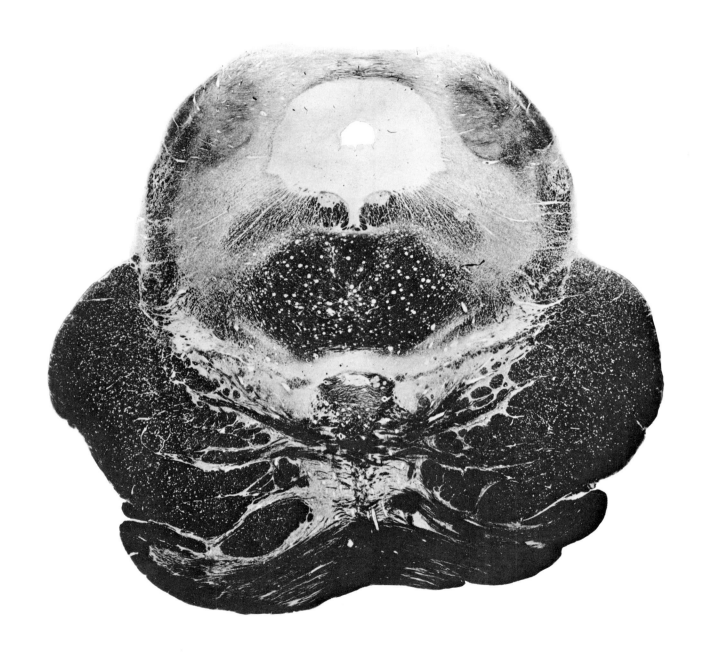

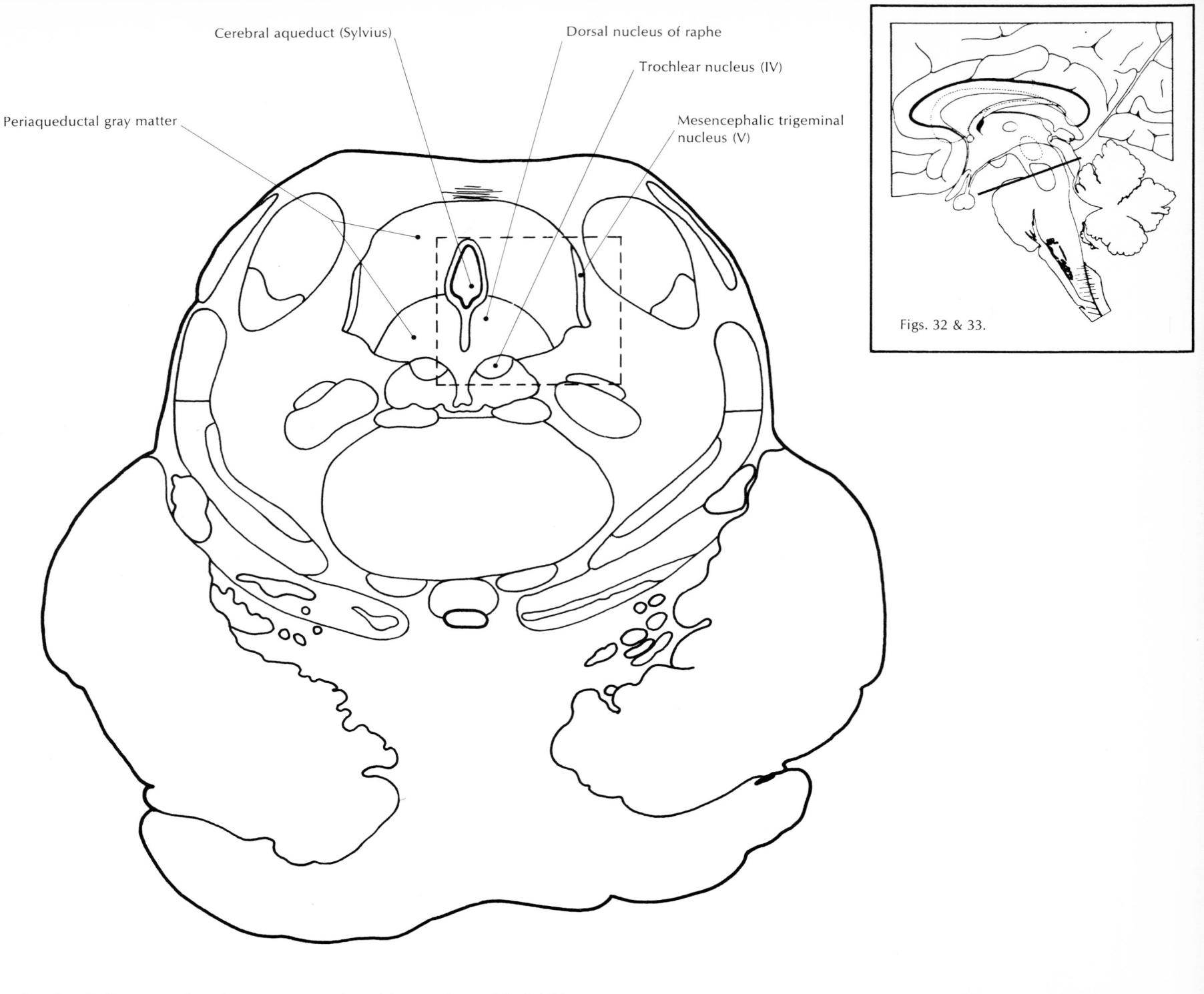

Periaqueductal gray matter

Cerebral aqueduct (Sylvius)

Dorsal nucleus of raphe

Trochlear nucleus (IV)

Mesencephalic trigeminal nucleus (V)

Figs. 32 & 33.

Figure 33. Midbrain: Inferior colliculus, detail of periaqueductal gray matter and trochlear nucleus—Nissl, 46X

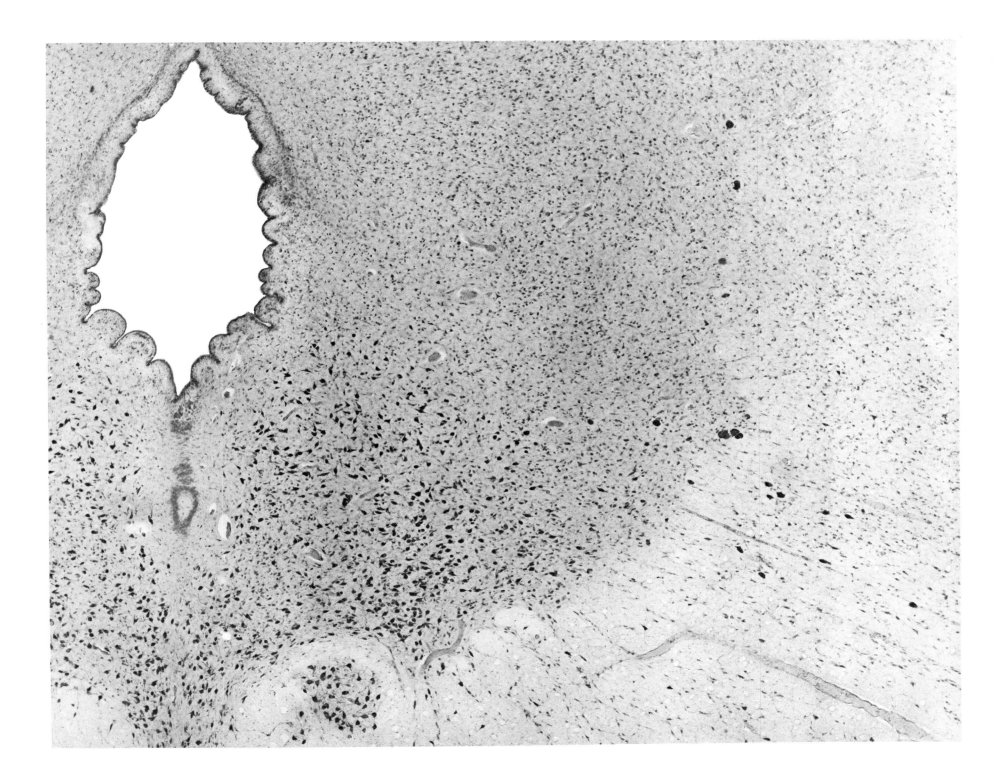

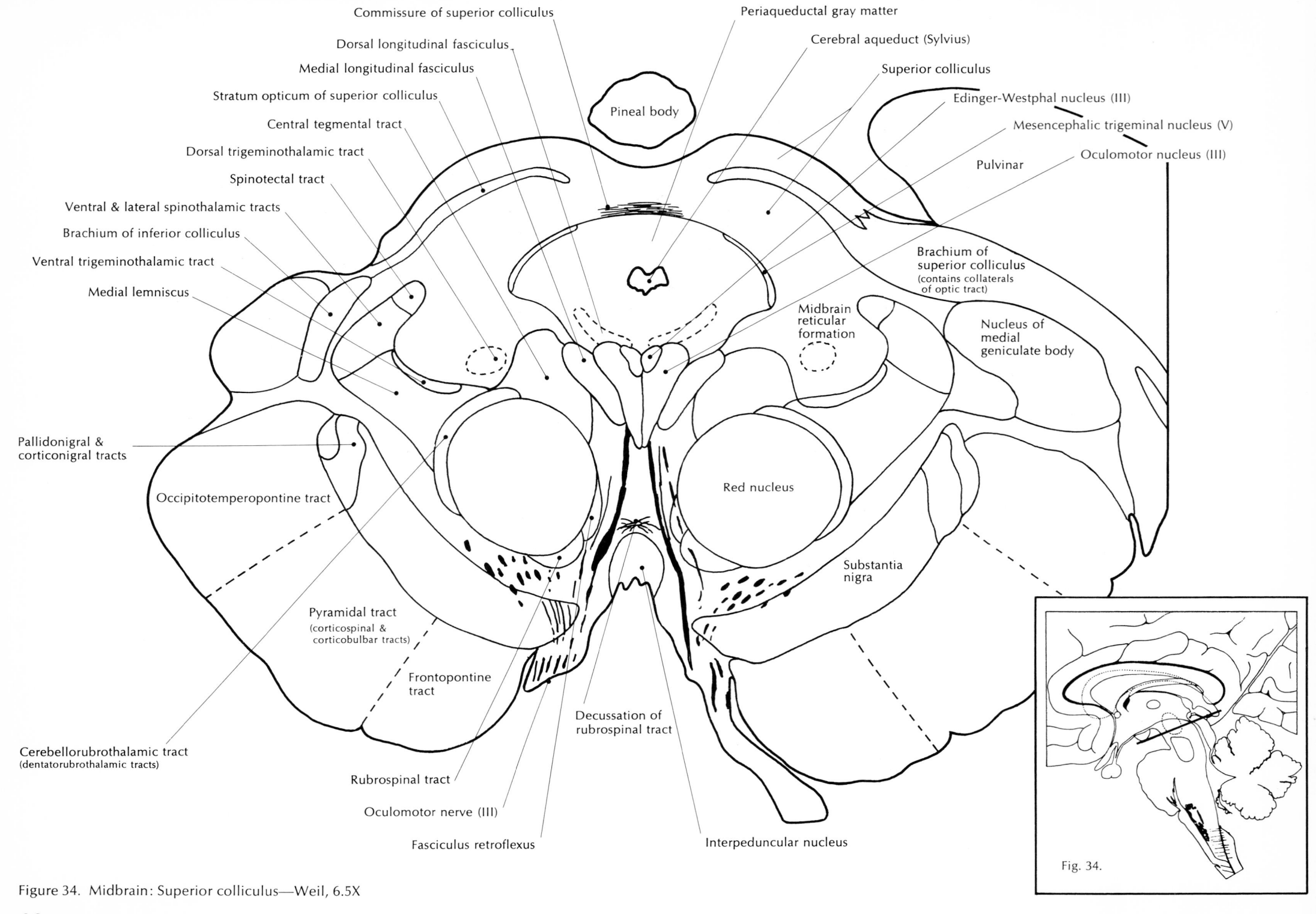

Figure 34. Midbrain: Superior colliculus—Weil, 6.5X

68

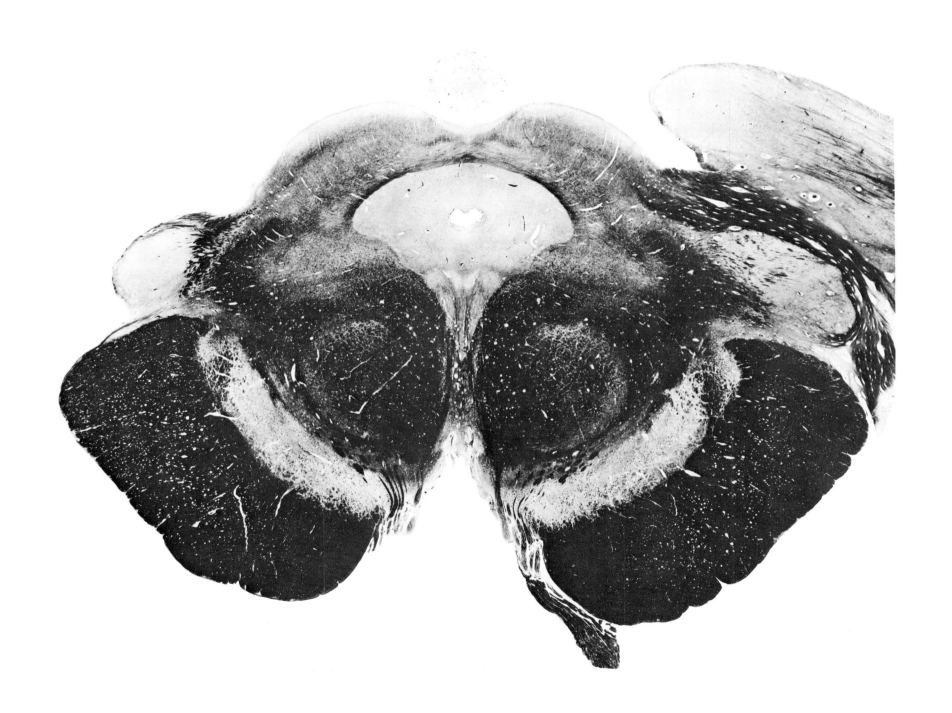

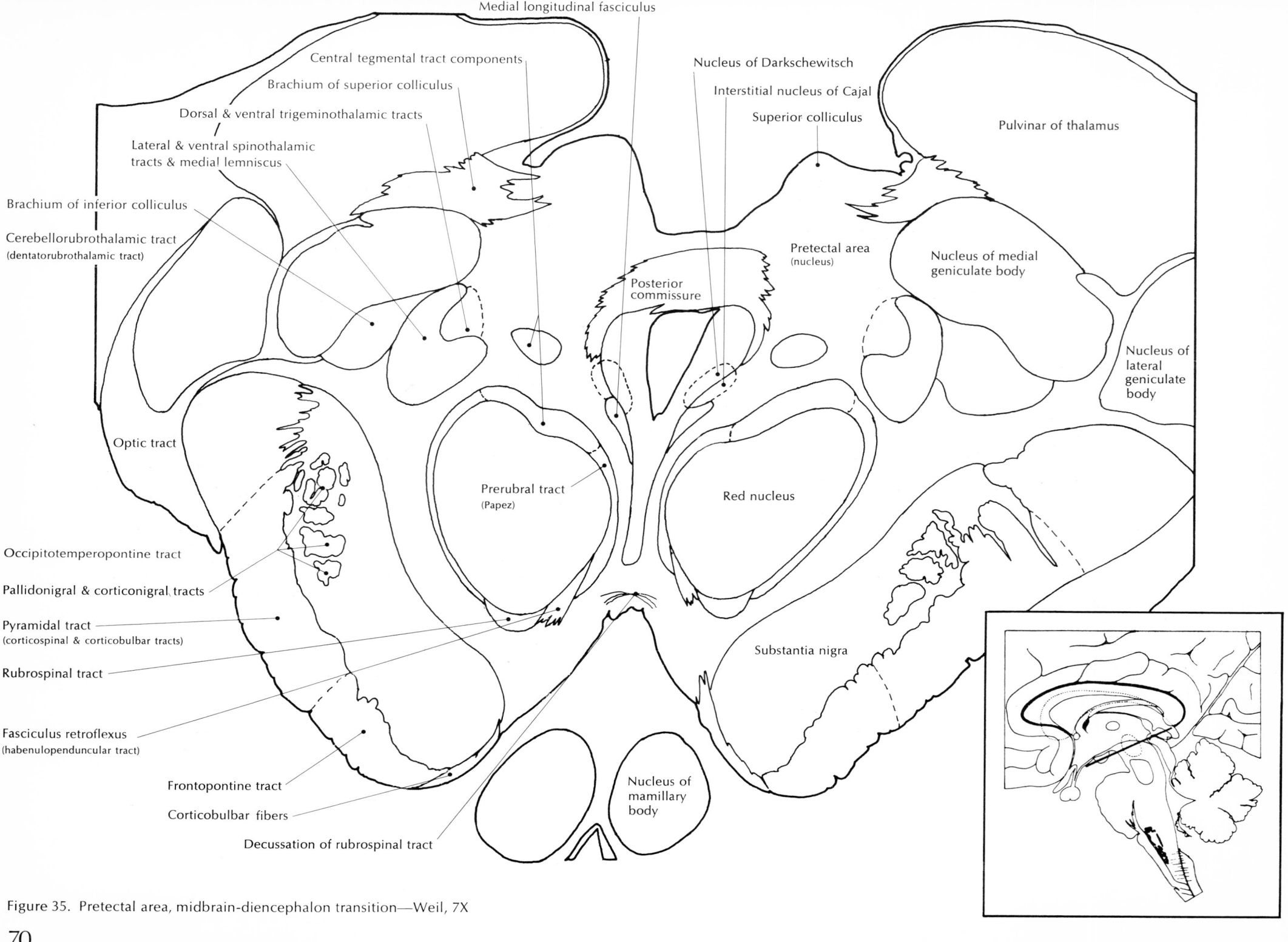

Medial longitudinal fasciculus

Central tegmental tract components

Brachium of superior colliculus

Dorsal & ventral trigeminothalamic tracts

Lateral & ventral spinothalamic tracts & medial lemniscus

Brachium of inferior colliculus

Cerebellorubrothalamic tract (dentatorubrothalamic tract)

Optic tract

Occipitotemperopontine tract

Pallidonigral & corticonigral tracts

Pyramidal tract (corticospinal & corticobulbar tracts)

Rubrospinal tract

Fasciculus retroflexus (habenulopenduncular tract)

Frontopontine tract

Corticobulbar fibers

Decussation of rubrospinal tract

Nucleus of Darkschewitsch

Interstitial nucleus of Cajal

Superior colliculus

Pulvinar of thalamus

Pretectal area (nucleus)

Posterior commissure

Nucleus of medial geniculate body

Nucleus of lateral geniculate body

Prerubral tract (Papez)

Red nucleus

Substantia nigra

Nucleus of mamillary body

Figure 35. Pretectal area, midbrain-diencephalon transition—Weil, 7X

70

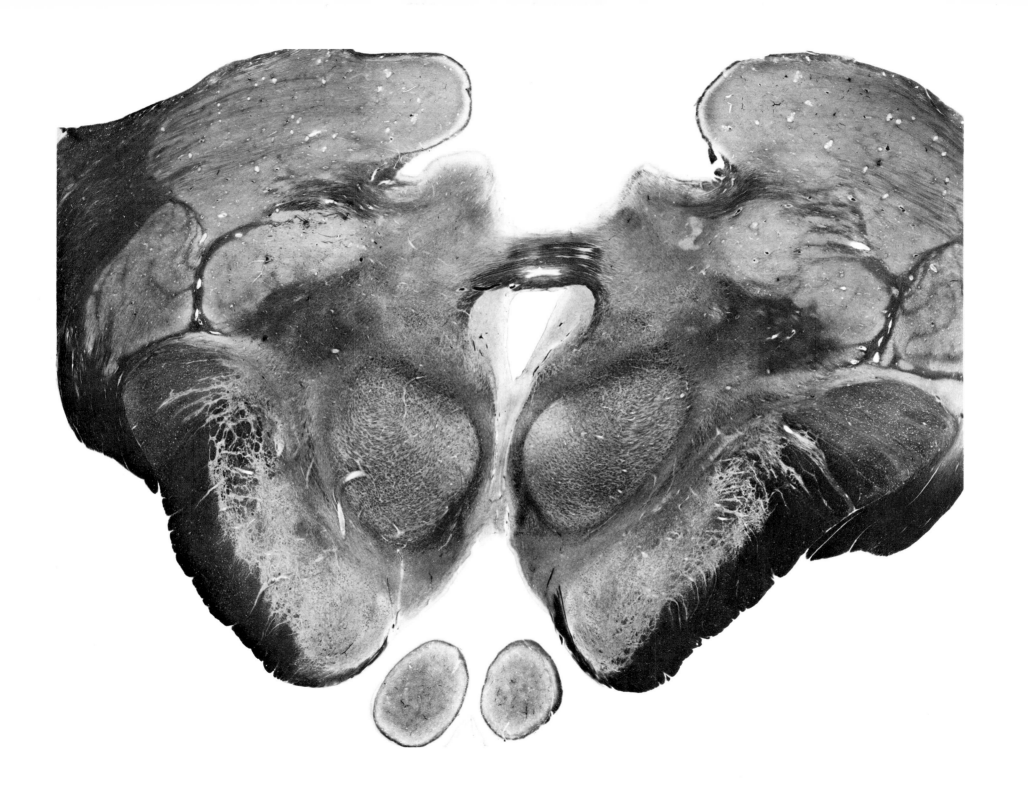

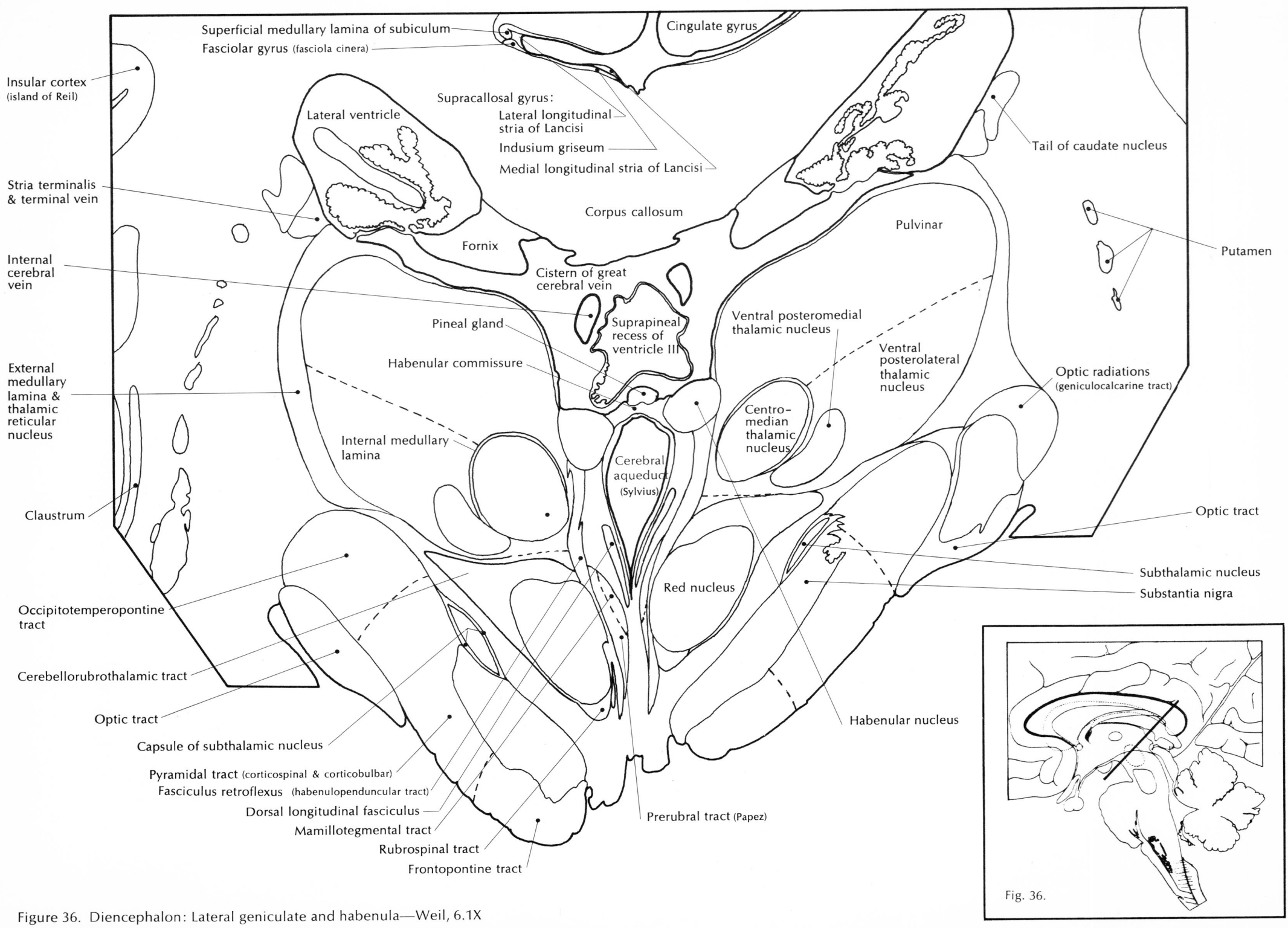

Insular cortex
(island of Reil)

Superficial medullary lamina of subiculum

Fasciolar gyrus (fasciola cinera)

Cingulate gyrus

Supracallosal gyrus:

Lateral longitudinal
stria of Lancisi

Indusium griseum

Medial longitudinal stria of Lancisi

Lateral ventricle

Tail of caudate nucleus

Stria terminalis
& terminal vein

Corpus callosum

Pulvinar

Putamen

Internal
cerebral
vein

Fornix

Cistern of great
cerebral vein

Ventral posteromedial
thalamic nucleus

External
medullary
lamina &
thalamic
reticular
nucleus

Pineal gland

Suprapineal
recess of
ventricle III

Habenular commissure

Ventral
posterolateral
thalamic
nucleus

Centro-
median
thalamic
nucleus

Optic radiations
(geniculocalcarine tract)

Internal medullary
lamina

Cerebral
aqueduct
(Sylvius)

Claustrum

Optic tract

Occipitotemperopontine
tract

Red nucleus

Subthalamic nucleus

Substantia nigra

Cerebellorubrothalamic tract

Optic tract

Capsule of subthalamic nucleus

Habenular nucleus

Pyramidal tract (corticospinal & corticobulbar)

Fasciculus retroflexus (habenulopenduncular tract)

Dorsal longitudinal fasciculus

Mamillotegmental tract

Prerubral tract (Papez)

Rubrospinal tract

Frontopontine tract

Fig. 36.

Figure 36. Diencephalon: Lateral geniculate and habenula—Weil, 6.1X

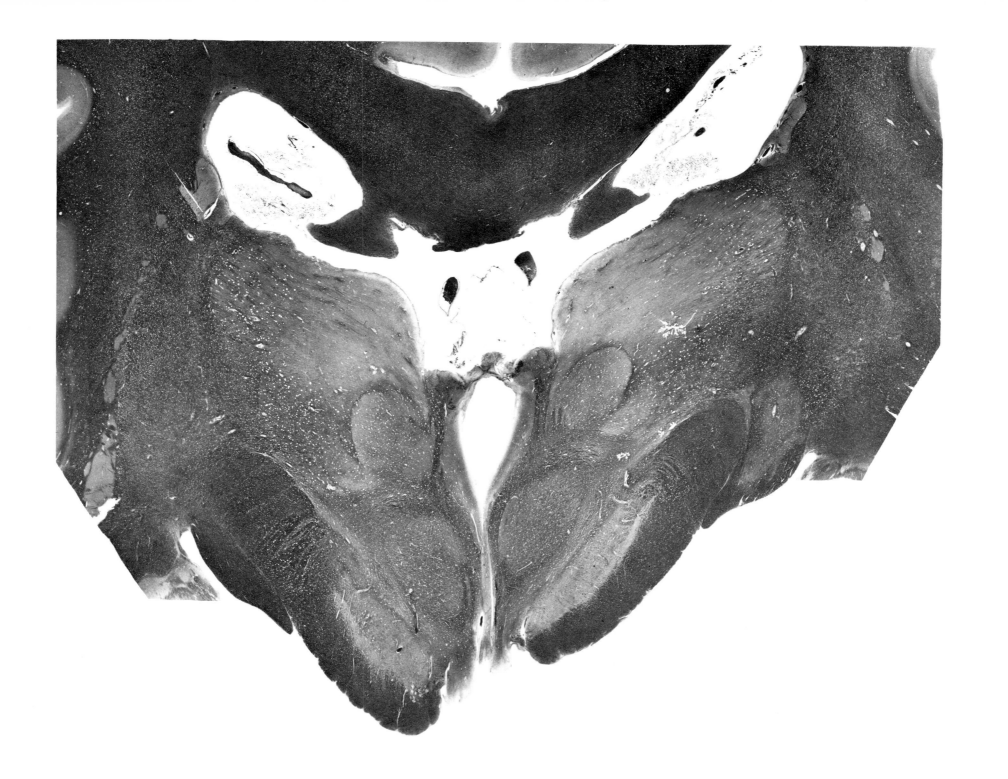

CORONAL SECTIONS OF THE BASAL GANGLIA AND DIENCEPHALON, INCLUDING HORIZONTAL SECTIONS OF THE BRAIN STEM

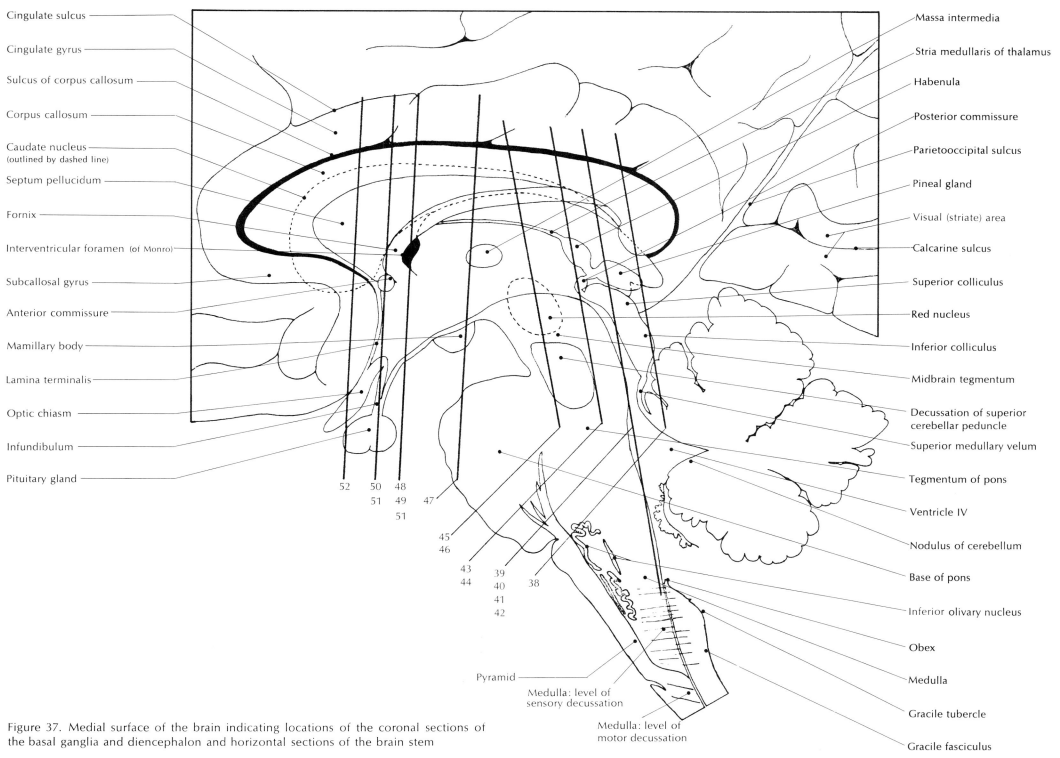

Cingulate sulcus

Cingulate gyrus

Sulcus of corpus callosum

Corpus callosum

Caudate nucleus
(outlined by dashed line)

Septum pellucidum

Fornix

Interventricular foramen (of Monro)

Subcallosal gyrus

Anterior commissure

Mamillary body

Lamina terminalis

Optic chiasm

Infundibulum

Pituitary gland

Massa intermedia

Stria medullaris of thalamus

Habenula

Posterior commissure

Parietooccipital sulcus

Pineal gland

Visual (striate) area

Calcarine sulcus

Superior colliculus

Red nucleus

Inferior colliculus

Midbrain tegmentum

Decussation of superior
cerebellar peduncle

Superior medullary velum

Tegmentum of pons

Ventricle IV

Nodulus of cerebellum

Base of pons

Inferior olivary nucleus

Obex

Medulla

Gracile tubercle

Gracile fasciculus

Pyramid

Medulla: level of
sensory decussation

Medulla: level of
motor decussation

52   50   48
    51   49   47
         51

45
46

43   39
44   40   38
     41
     42

Figure 37. Medial surface of the brain indicating locations of the coronal sections of
the basal ganglia and diencephalon and horizontal sections of the brain stem

75

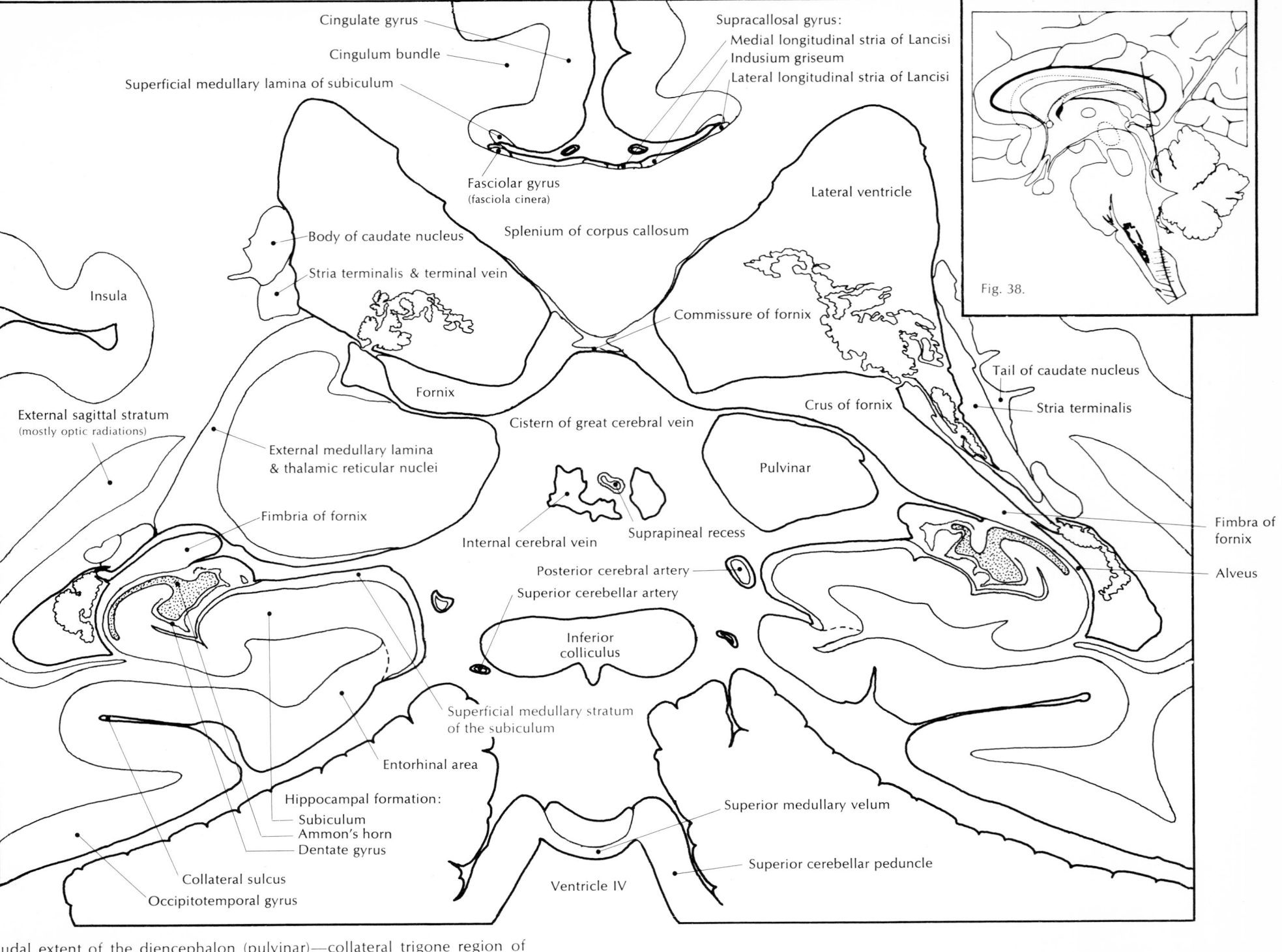

Figure 38. Caudal extent of the diencephalon (pulvinar)—collateral trigone region of
lateral ventricle (note continuity of the alevus, fimbria, and fornix fiber system)—Weil, 4X

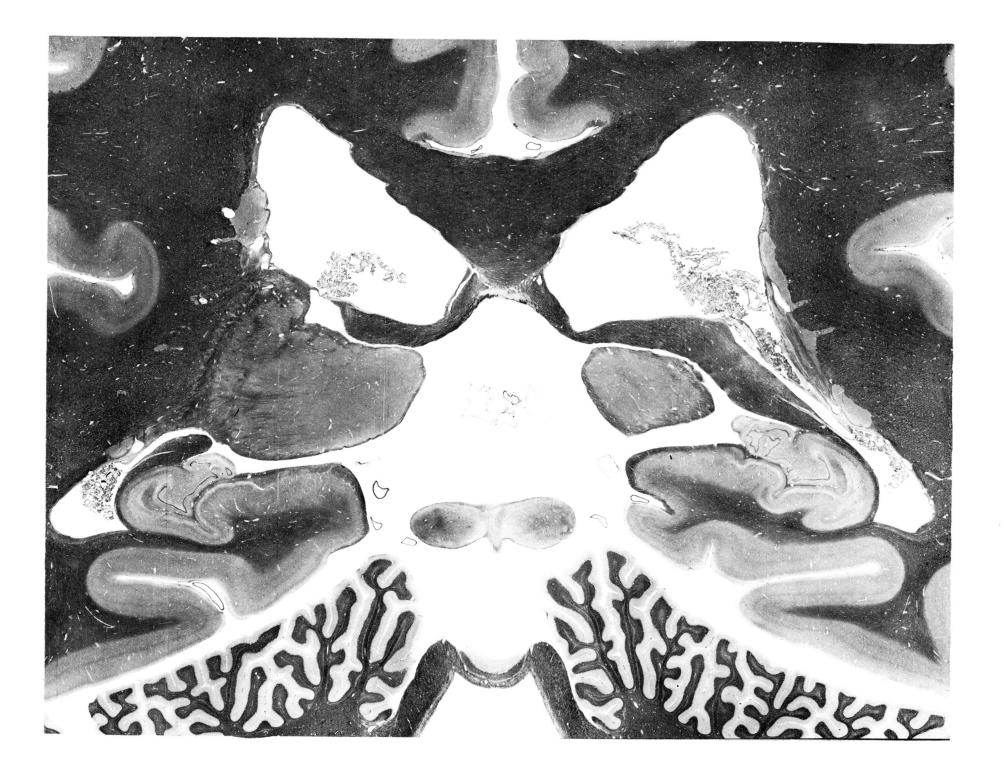

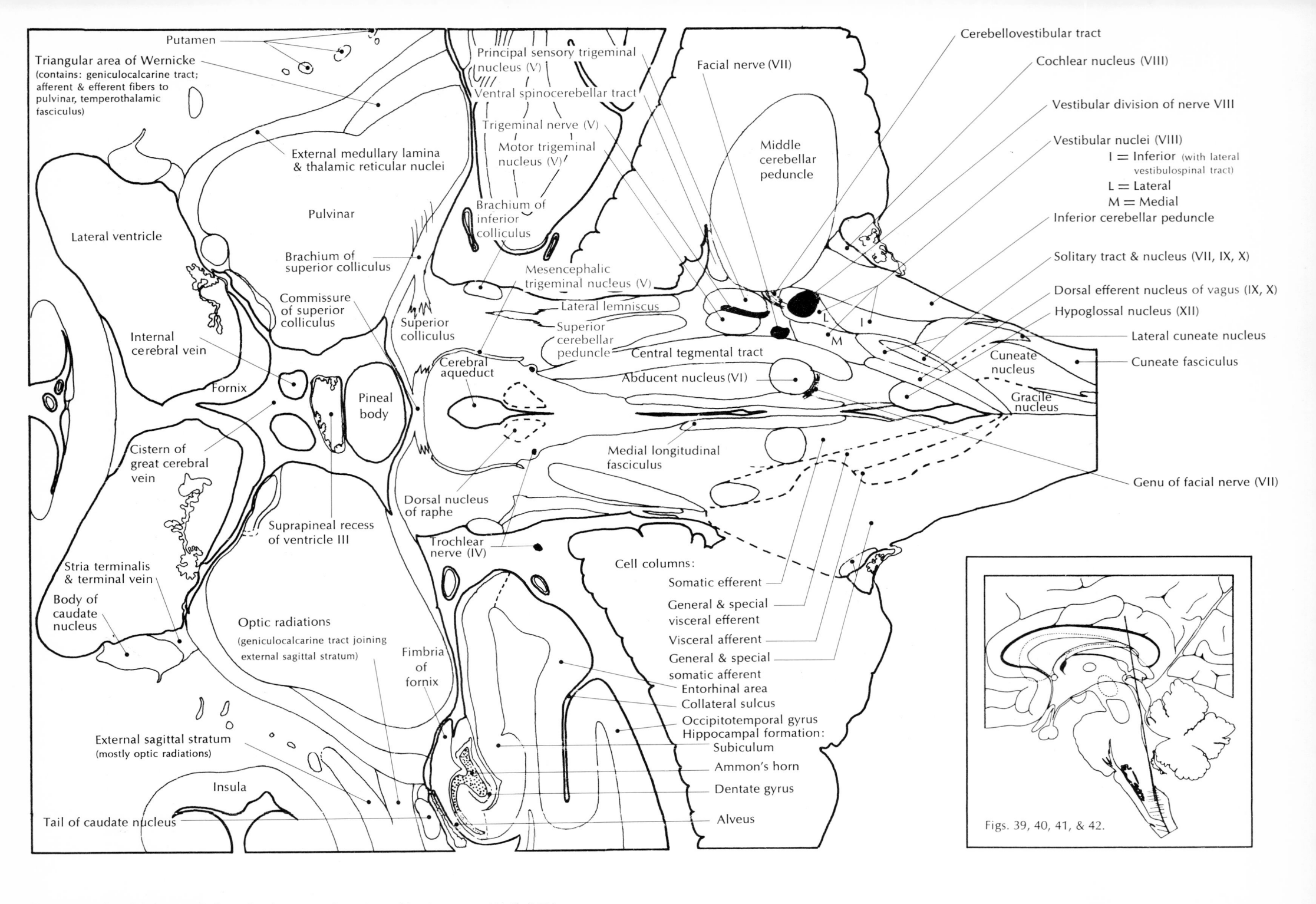

Putamen

Triangular area of Wernicke
(contains: geniculocalcarine tract;
afferent & efferent fibers to
pulvinar, temperothalamic
fasciculus)

External medullary lamina
& thalamic reticular nuclei

Pulvinar

Lateral ventricle

Brachium of
superior colliculus

Commissure
of superior
colliculus

Internal
cerebral vein

Fornix

Pineal
body

Cistern of
great cerebral
vein

Suprapineal recess
of ventricle III

Stria terminalis
& terminal vein

Body of
caudate
nucleus

Optic radiations
(geniculocalcarine tract joining
external sagittal stratum)

External sagittal stratum
(mostly optic radiations)

Insula

Tail of caudate nucleus

Principal sensory trigeminal
nucleus (V)

Ventral spinocerebellar tract

Trigeminal nerve (V)

Motor trigeminal
nucleus (V)

Brachium of
inferior
colliculus

Mesencephalic
trigeminal nucleus (V)

Lateral lemniscus

Superior
colliculus

Superior
cerebellar
peduncle

Cerebral
aqueduct

Dorsal nucleus
of raphe

Trochlear
nerve (IV)

Fimbria
of
fornix

Facial nerve (VII)

Middle
cerebellar
peduncle

Central tegmental tract

Abducent nucleus (VI)

Medial longitudinal
fasciculus

Cell columns:

Somatic efferent

General & special
visceral efferent

Visceral afferent

General & special
somatic afferent

Entorhinal area

Collateral sulcus

Occipitotemporal gyrus

Hippocampal formation:
Subiculum

Ammon's horn

Dentate gyrus

Alveus

Cerebellovestibular tract

Cochlear nucleus (VIII)

Vestibular division of nerve VIII

Vestibular nuclei (VIII)
I = Inferior (with lateral
vestibulospinal tract)
L = Lateral
M = Medial
Inferior cerebellar peduncle

Solitary tract & nucleus (VII, IX, X)

Dorsal efferent nucleus of vagus (IX, X)

Hypoglossal nucleus (XII)

Lateral cuneate nucleus

Cuneate
nucleus

Cuneate fasciculus

Gracile
nucleus

Genu of facial nerve (VII)

L   I

M

Figs. 39, 40, 41, & 42.

Figure 39. Caudal diencephalon plus horizontal section of brain stem—Weil. 2.3X

78

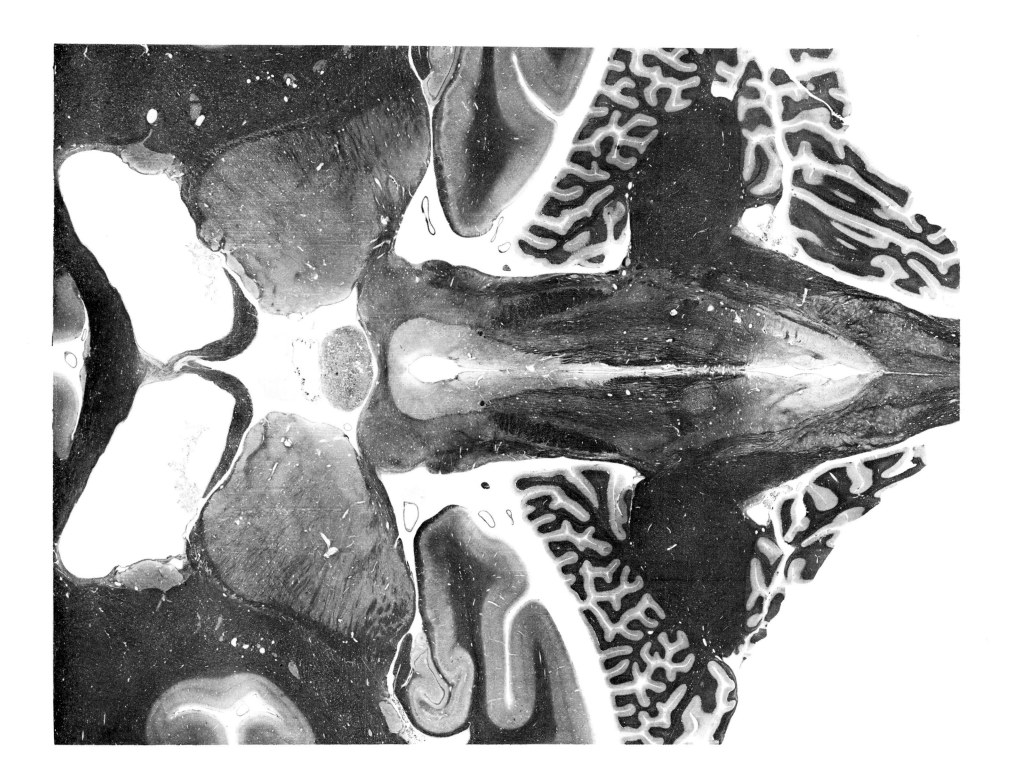

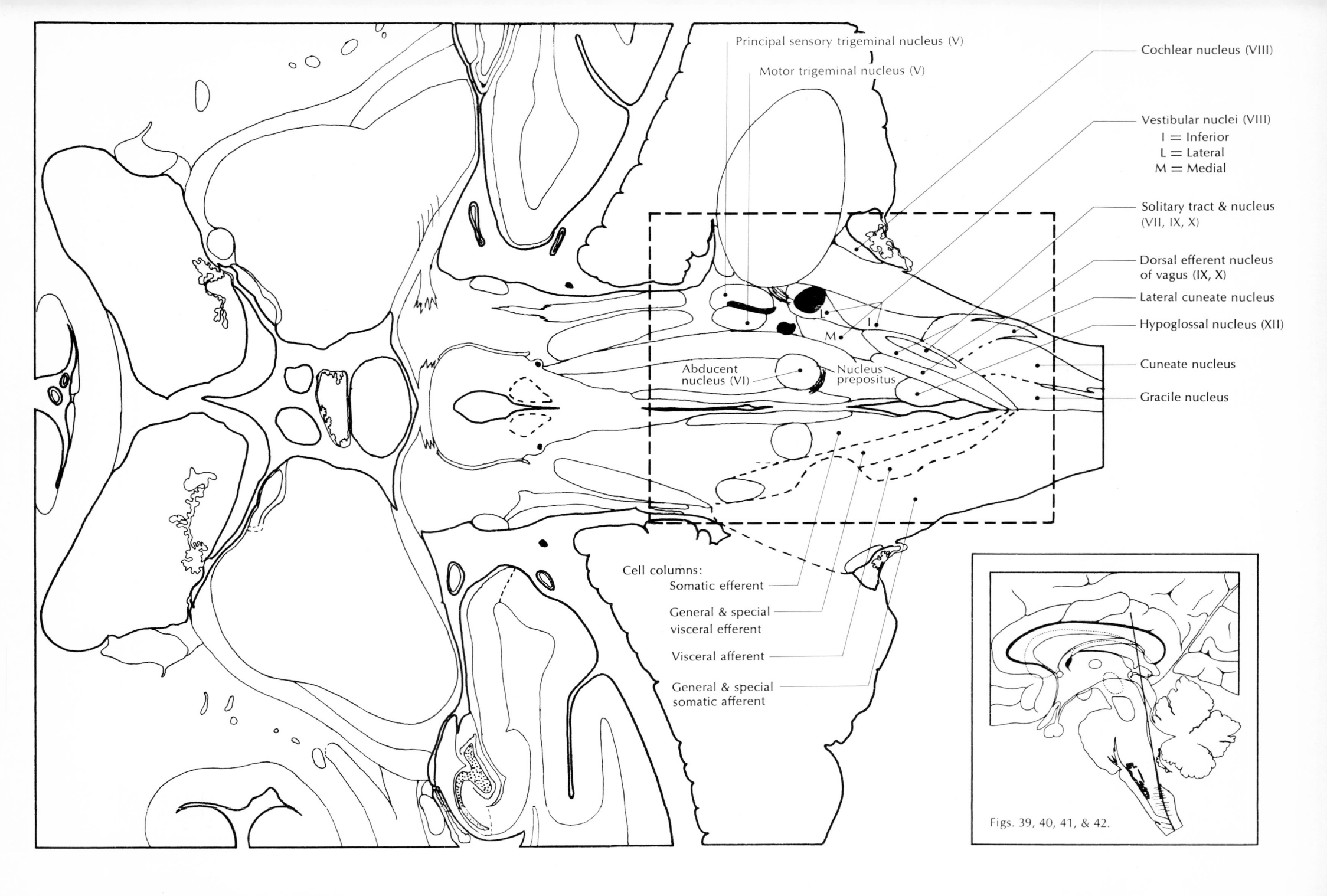

Principal sensory trigeminal nucleus (V)

Motor trigeminal nucleus (V)

Cochlear nucleus (VIII)

Vestibular nuclei (VIII)
I = Inferior
L = Lateral
M = Medial

Solitary tract & nucleus (VII, IX, X)

Dorsal efferent nucleus of vagus (IX, X)

Lateral cuneate nucleus

Hypoglossal nucleus (XII)

Cuneate nucleus

Gracile nucleus

Abducent nucleus (VI)

Nucleus prepositus

Cell columns:
Somatic efferent

General & special visceral efferent

Visceral afferent

General & special somatic afferent

Figs. 39, 40, 41, & 42.

Figure 40. Cell columns and functional components of cranial nerve nuclei in the pons and medulla—Nissl, 10X

80

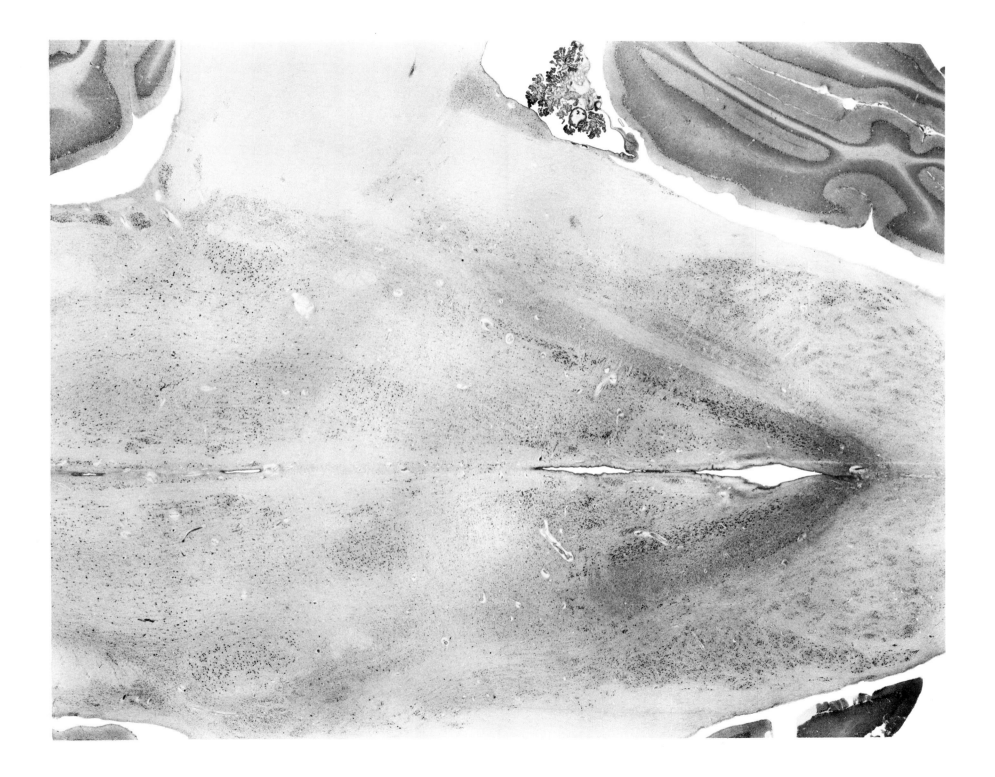

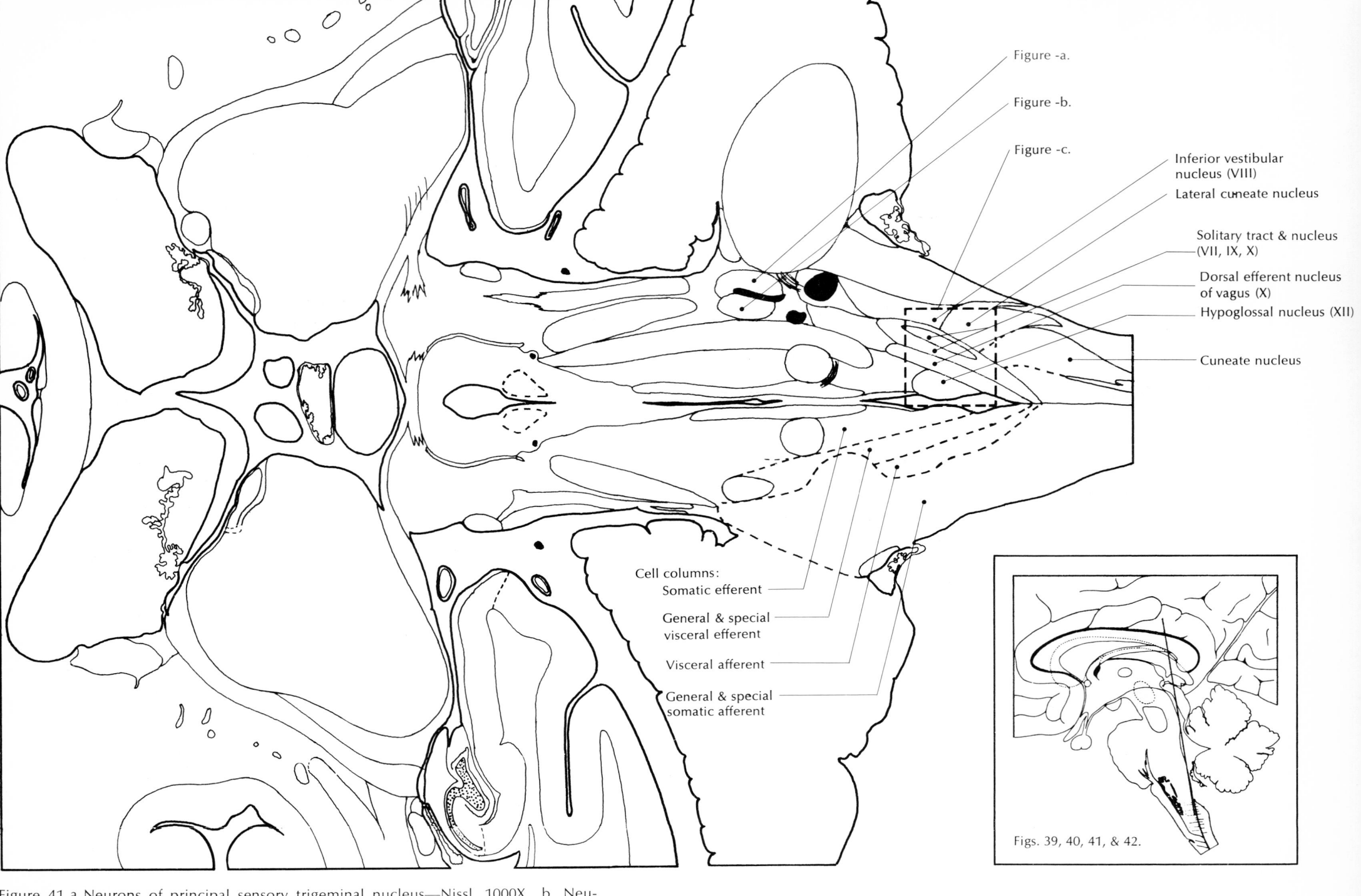

Figure -a.

Figure -b.

Figure -c.

Inferior vestibular nucleus (VIII)

Lateral cuneate nucleus

Solitary tract & nucleus (VII, IX, X)

Dorsal efferent nucleus of vagus (X)

Hypoglossal nucleus (XII)

Cuneate nucleus

Cell columns:
Somatic efferent

General & special visceral efferent

Visceral afferent

General & special somatic afferent

Figs. 39, 40, 41, & 42.

Figure 41 a. Neurons of principal sensory trigeminal nucleus—Nissl, 1000X b. Neurons of motor trigeminal nucleus—Nissl, 1000X c. Detail of cell columns and functional components of cranial nerve nuclei of the medulla—Nissl, 40X

82

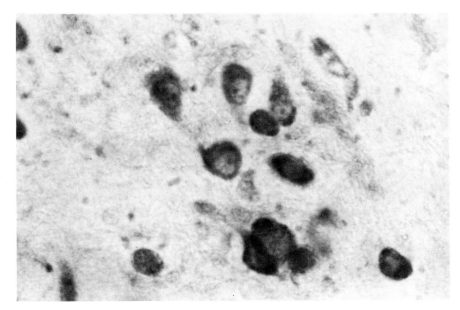

a.

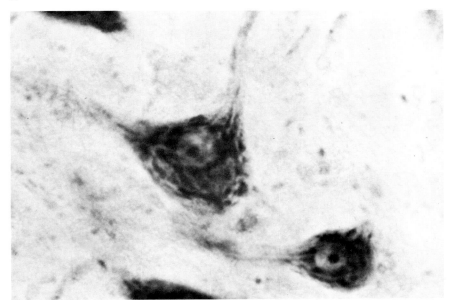

b.

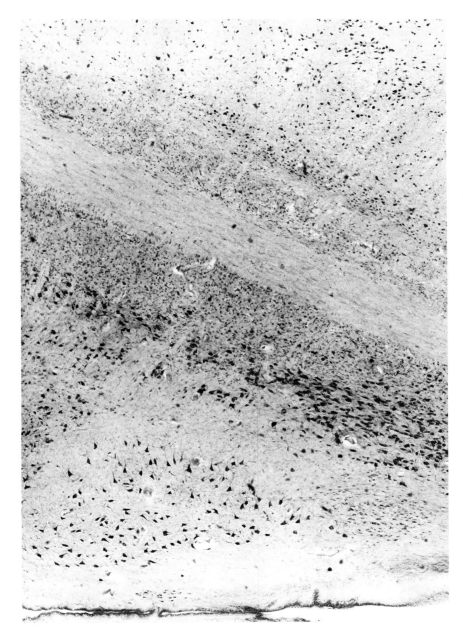

c.

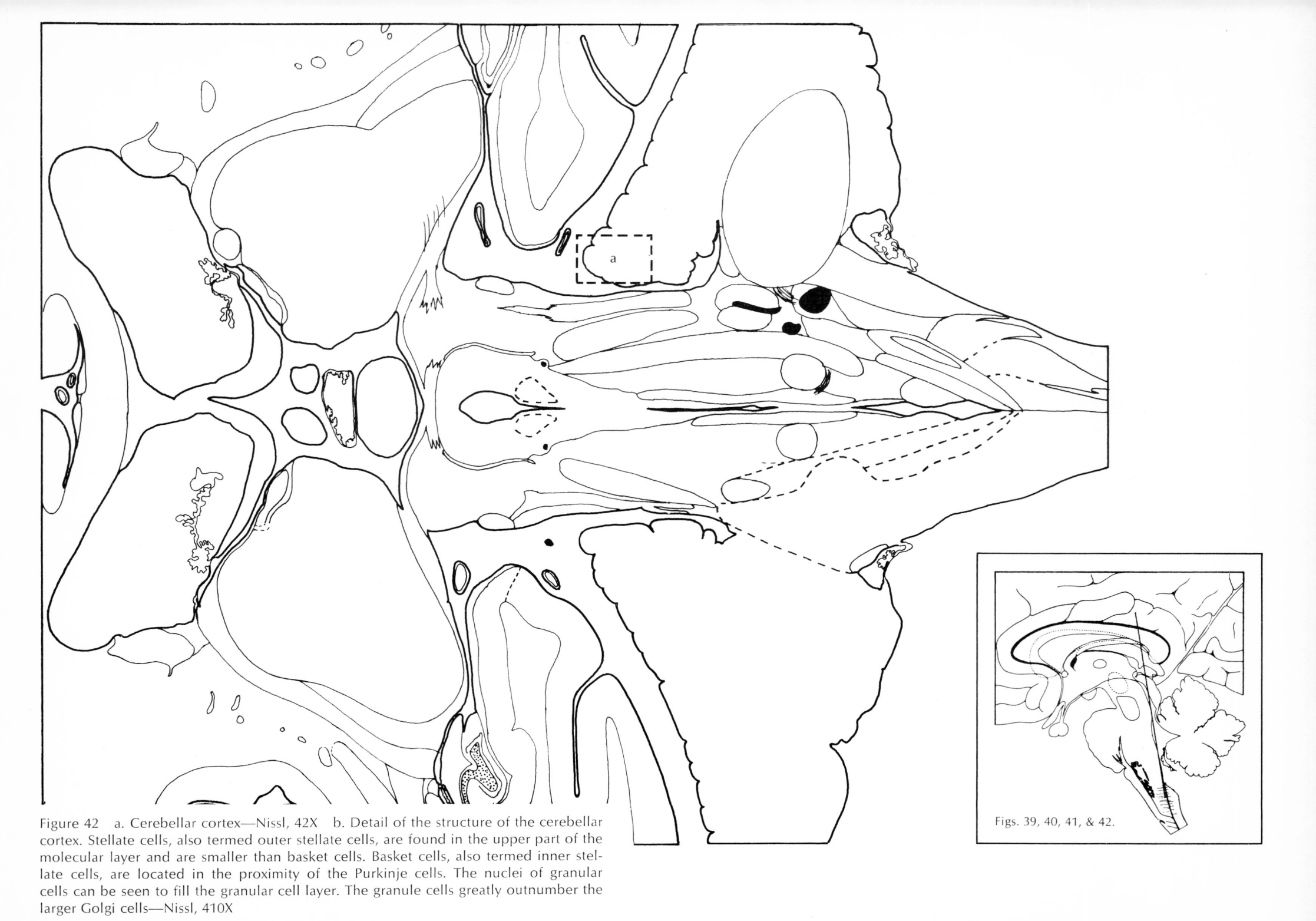

Figure 42   a. Cerebellar cortex—Nissl, 42X   b. Detail of the structure of the cerebellar
cortex. Stellate cells, also termed outer stellate cells, are found in the upper part of the
molecular layer and are smaller than basket cells. Basket cells, also termed inner stellate cells, are located in the proximity of the Purkinje cells. The nuclei of granular
cells can be seen to fill the granular cell layer. The granule cells greatly outnumber the
larger Golgi cells—Nissl, 410X

Figs. 39, 40, 41, & 42.

84

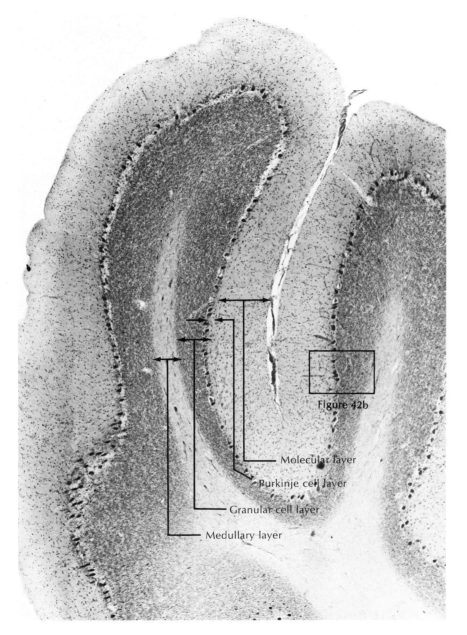

Molecular layer

Purkinje cell layer

Granular cell layer

Medullary layer

Figure 42b

a.

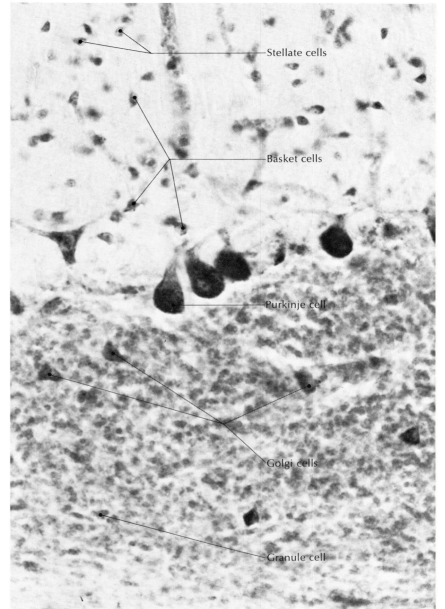

Stellate cells

Basket cells

Purkinje cell

Golgi cells

Granule cell

b.

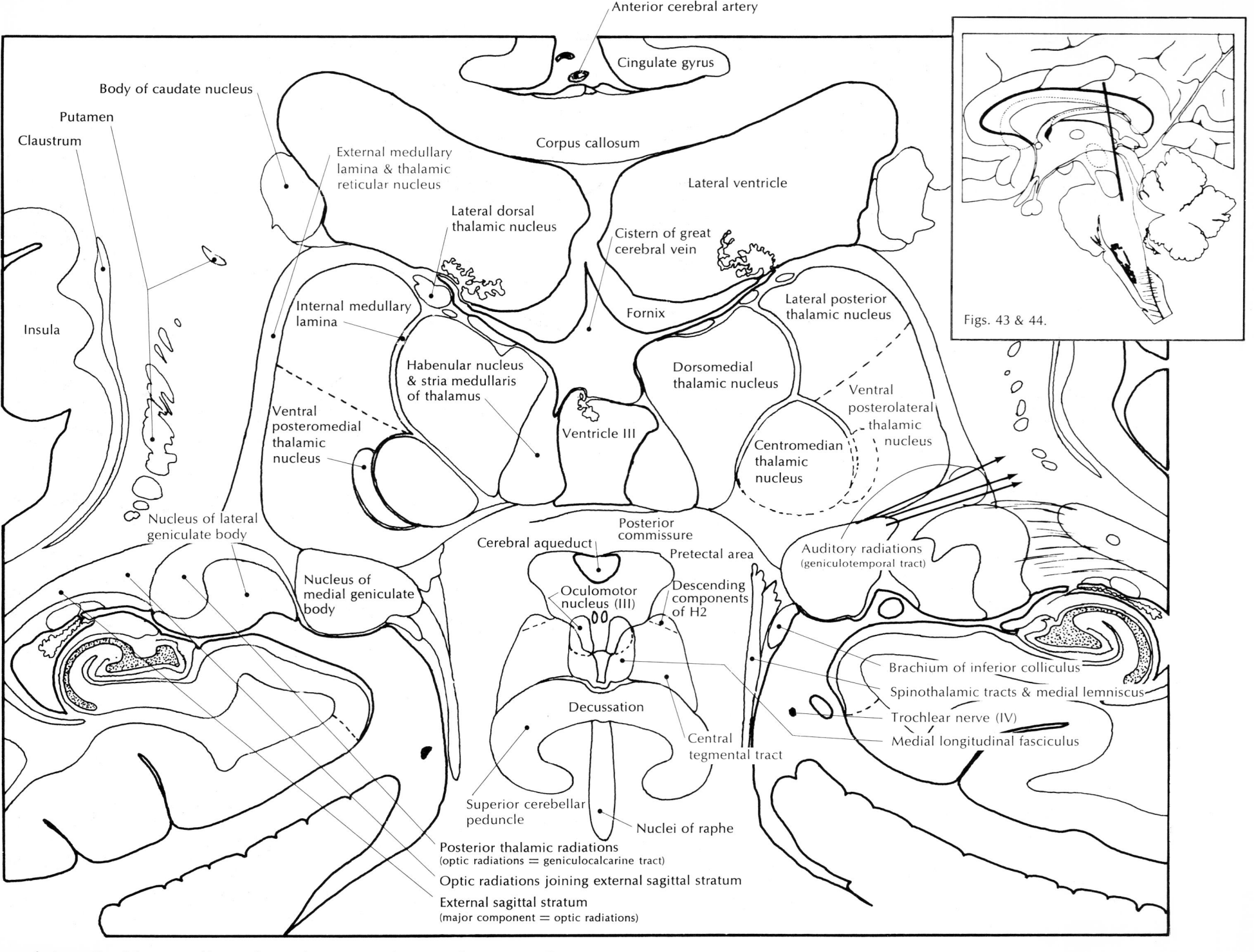

Figure 43. Diencephalon—Caudal extent of lenticular nucleus at posterior commissure — Weil, 4X

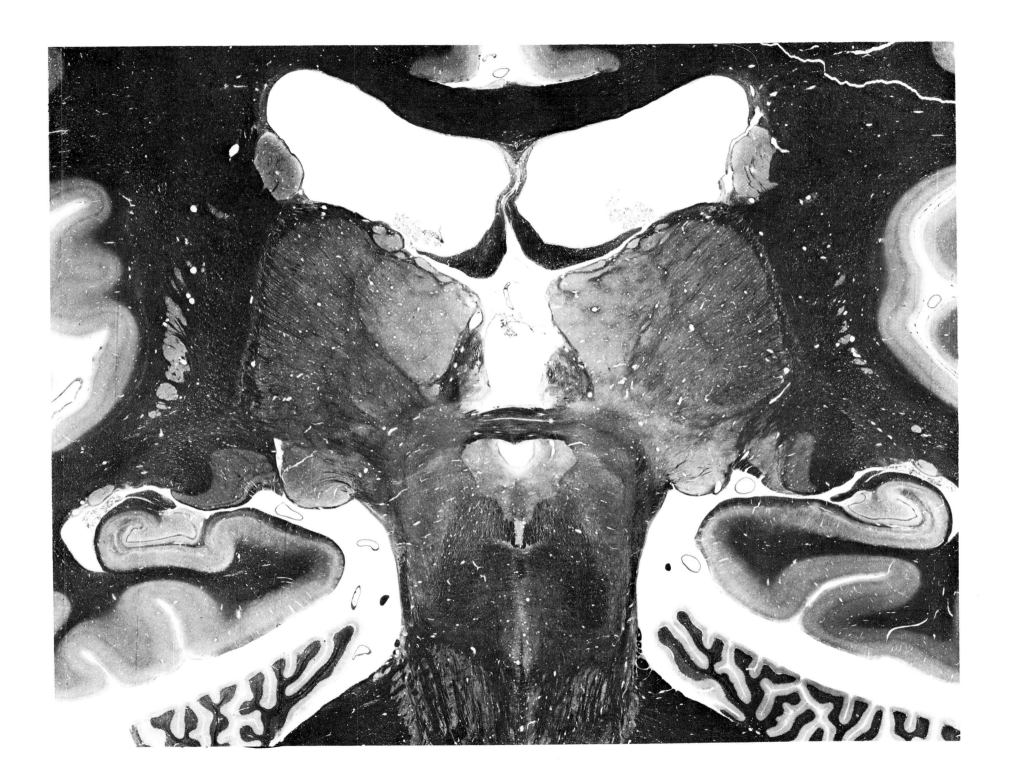

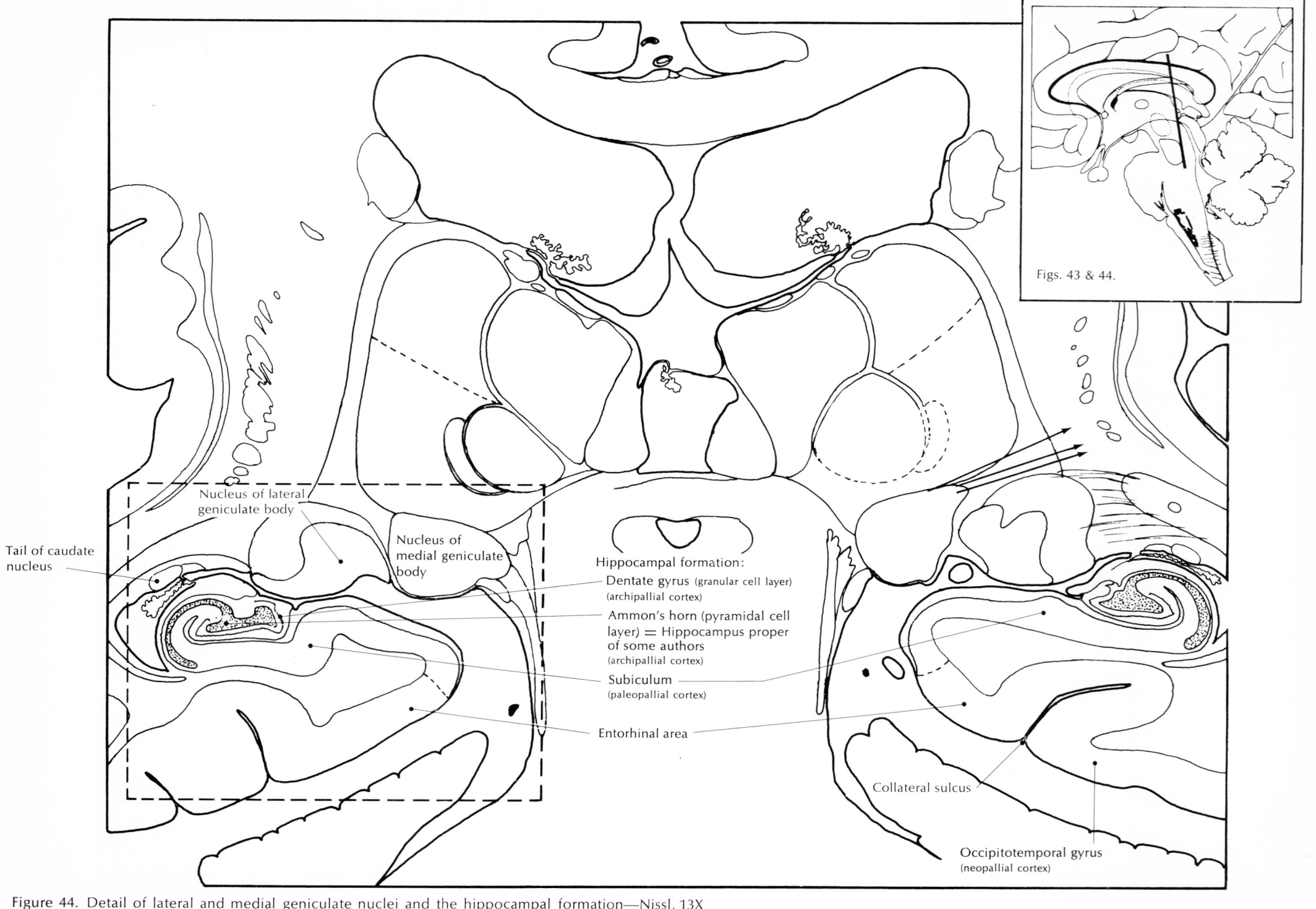

Figure 44. Detail of lateral and medial geniculate nuclei and the hippocampal formation—Nissl, 13X

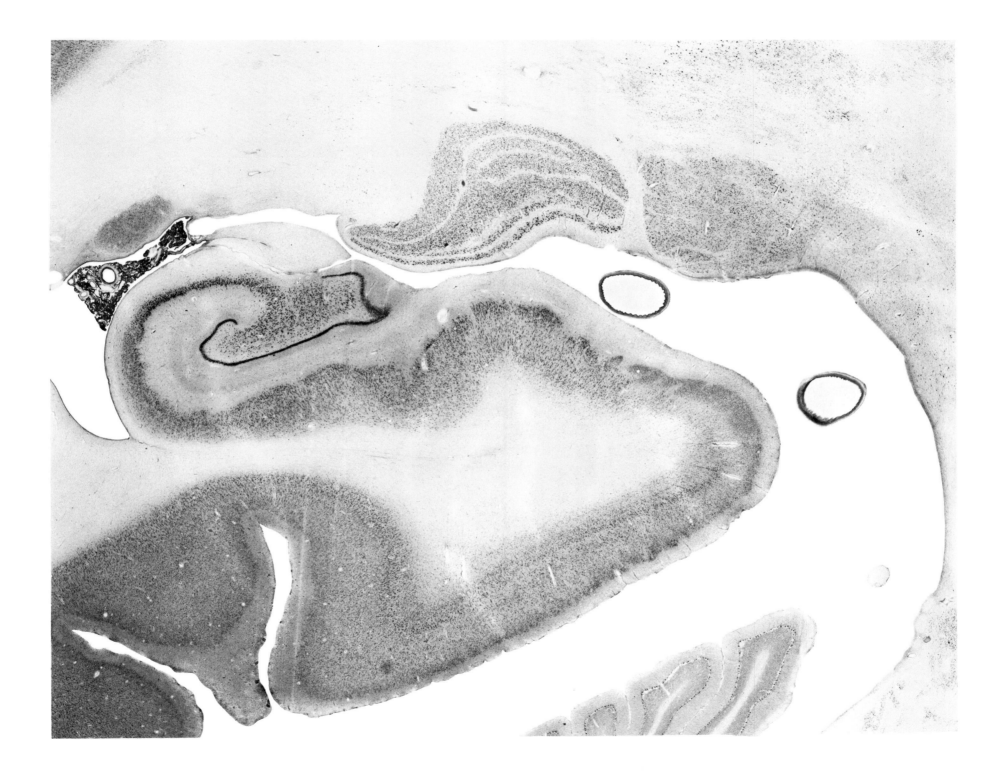

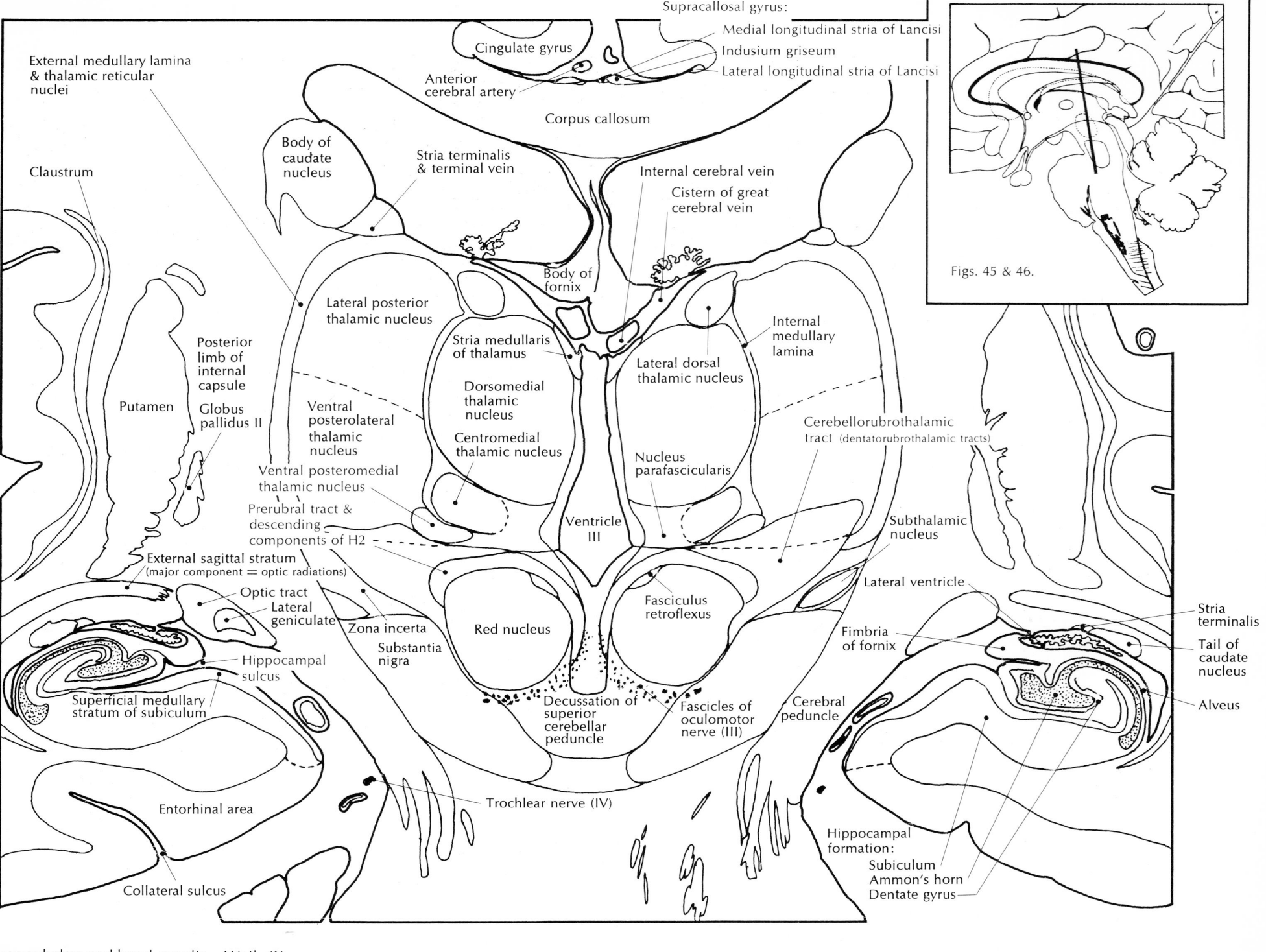

Figure 45. Diencephalon and basal ganglia—Weil, 4X

90

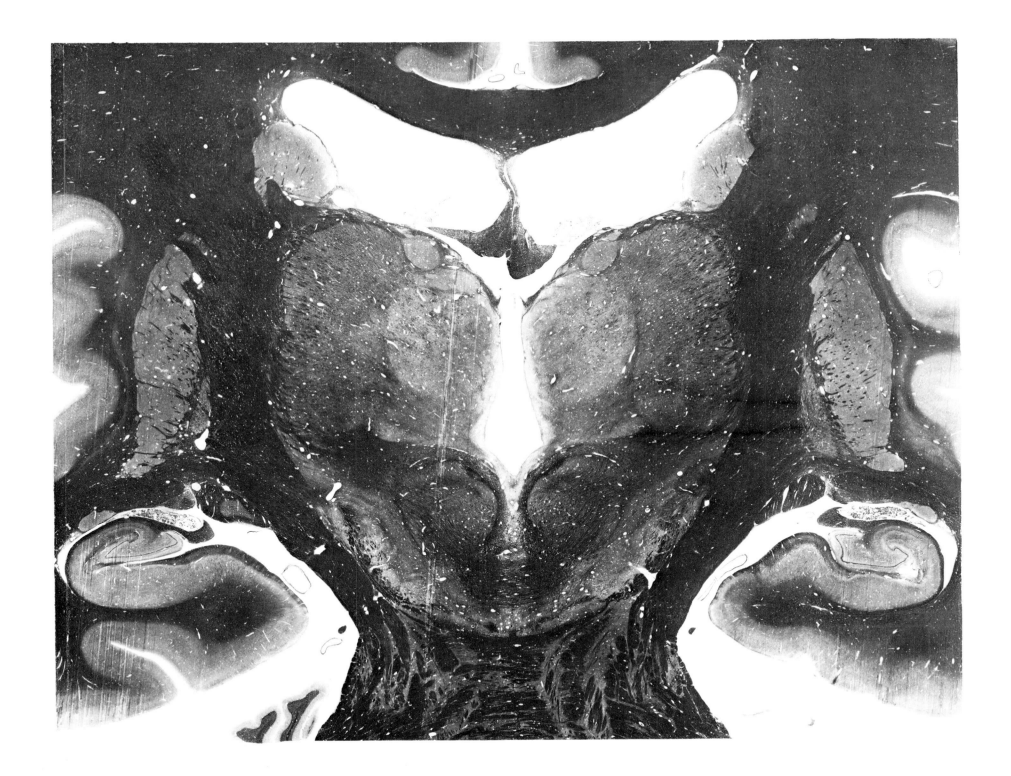

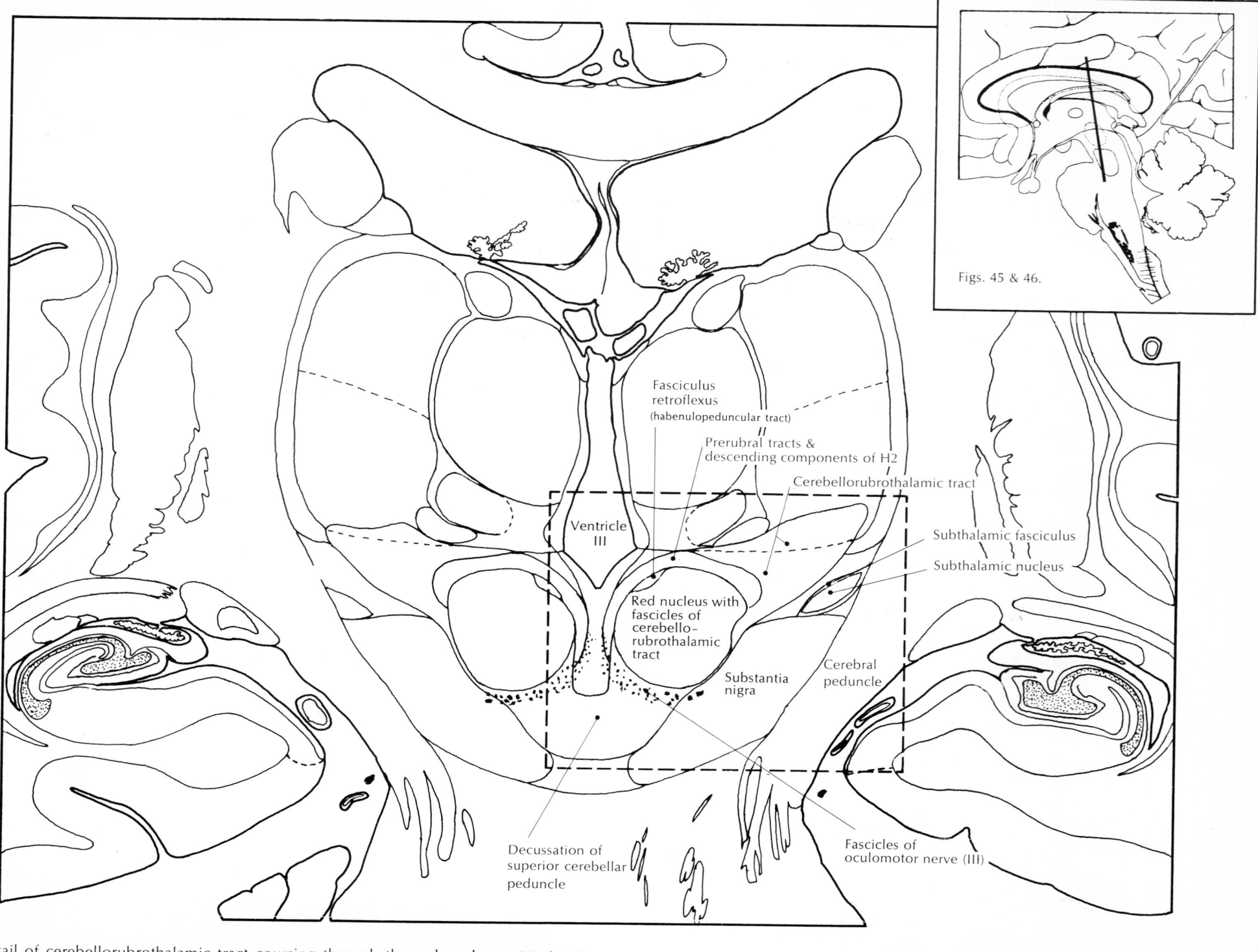

Figs. 45 & 46.

Fasciculus
retroflexus
(habenulopeduncular tract)

Prerubral tracts &
descending components of H2

Cerebellorubrothalamic tract

Subthalamic fasciculus

Subthalamic nucleus

Ventricle
III

Red nucleus with
fascicles of
cerebello-
rubrothalamic
tract

Substantia
nigra

Cerebral
peduncle

Decussation of
superior cerebellar
peduncle

Fascicles of
oculomotor nerve (III)

Figure 46. Detail of cerebellorubrothalamic tract coursing through the red nucleus— Weil, 13X

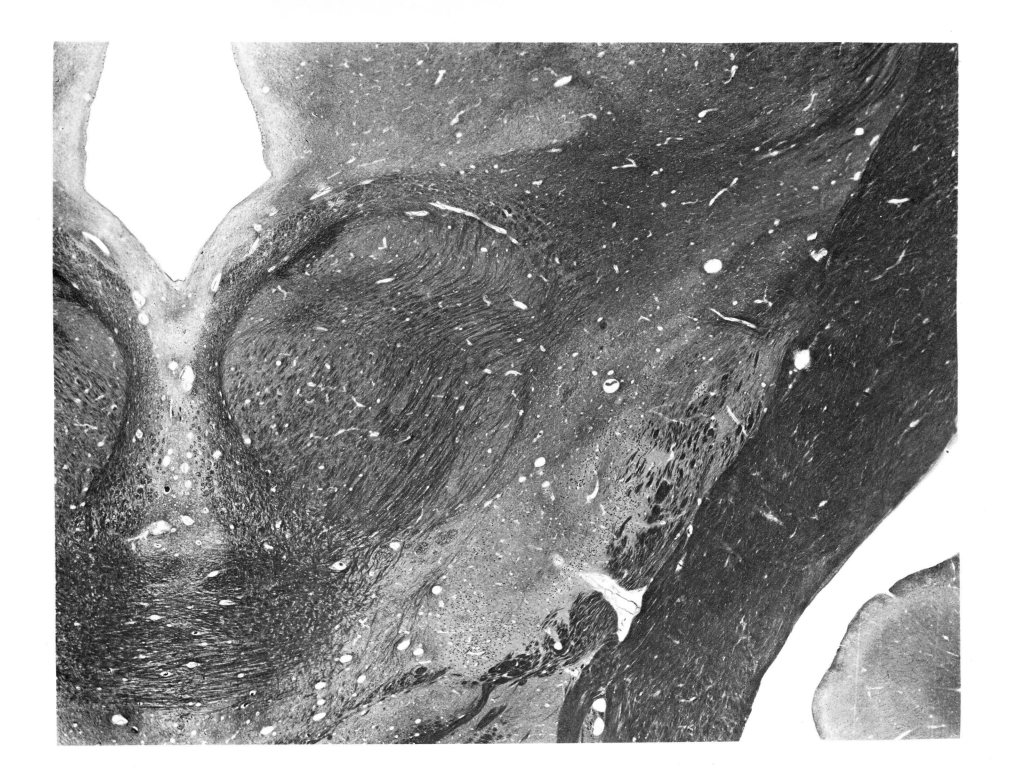

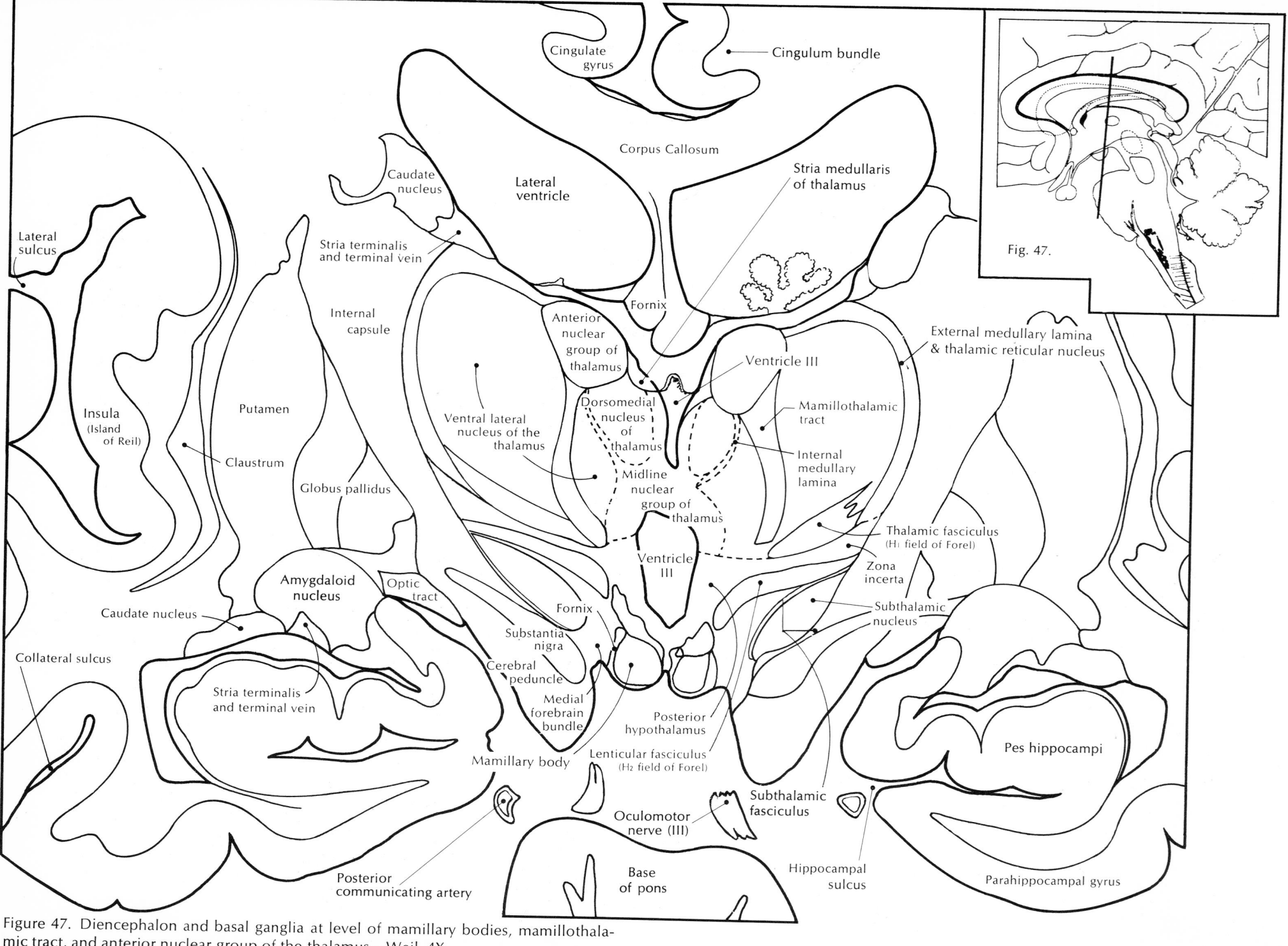

Figure 47. Diencephalon and basal ganglia at level of mamillary bodies, mamillothalamic tract, and anterior nuclear group of the thalamus—Weil, 4X

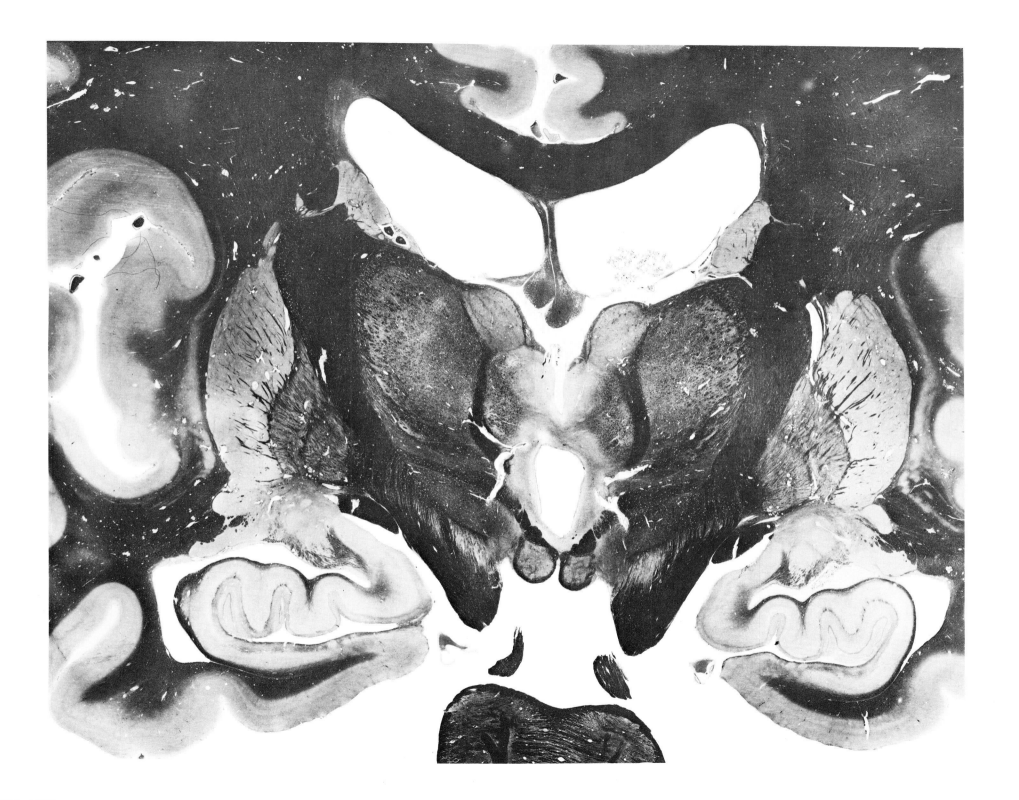

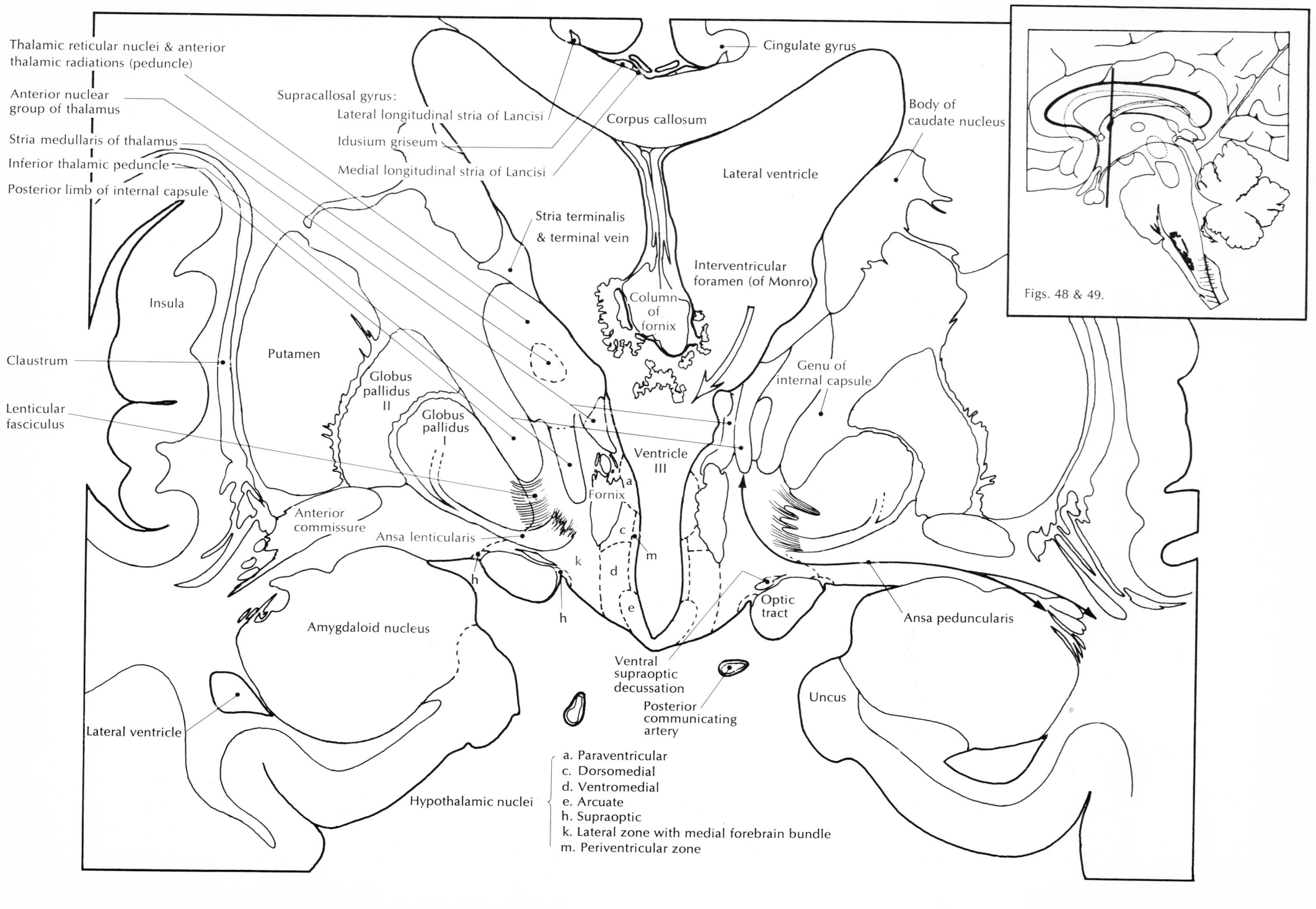

Thalamic reticular nuclei & anterior thalamic radiations (peduncle)

Anterior nuclear group of thalamus

Stria medullaris of thalamus

Inferior thalamic peduncle

Posterior limb of internal capsule

Supracallosal gyrus:

Lateral longitudinal stria of Lancisi

Idusium griseum

Medial longitudinal stria of Lancisi

Cingulate gyrus

Corpus callosum

Body of caudate nucleus

Lateral ventricle

Stria terminalis & terminal vein

Interventricular foramen (of Monro)

Figs. 48 & 49.

Insula

Column of fornix

Claustrum

Putamen

Globus pallidus II

Globus pallidus I

Genu of internal capsule

Lenticular fasciculus

Ventricle III

Fornix

a

Anterior commissure

Ansa lenticularis

c

m

k

d

h

e

h

Optic tract

Ansa peduncularis

Amygdaloid nucleus

Ventral supraoptic decussation

Posterior communicating artery

Uncus

Lateral ventricle

Hypothalamic nuclei

a. Paraventricular
c. Dorsomedial
d. Ventromedial
e. Arcuate
h. Supraoptic
k. Lateral zone with medial forebrain bundle
m. Periventricular zone

Figure 48. Basal ganglia and rostral diencephalon, tuberal region of hypothalamus—Weil, 4X

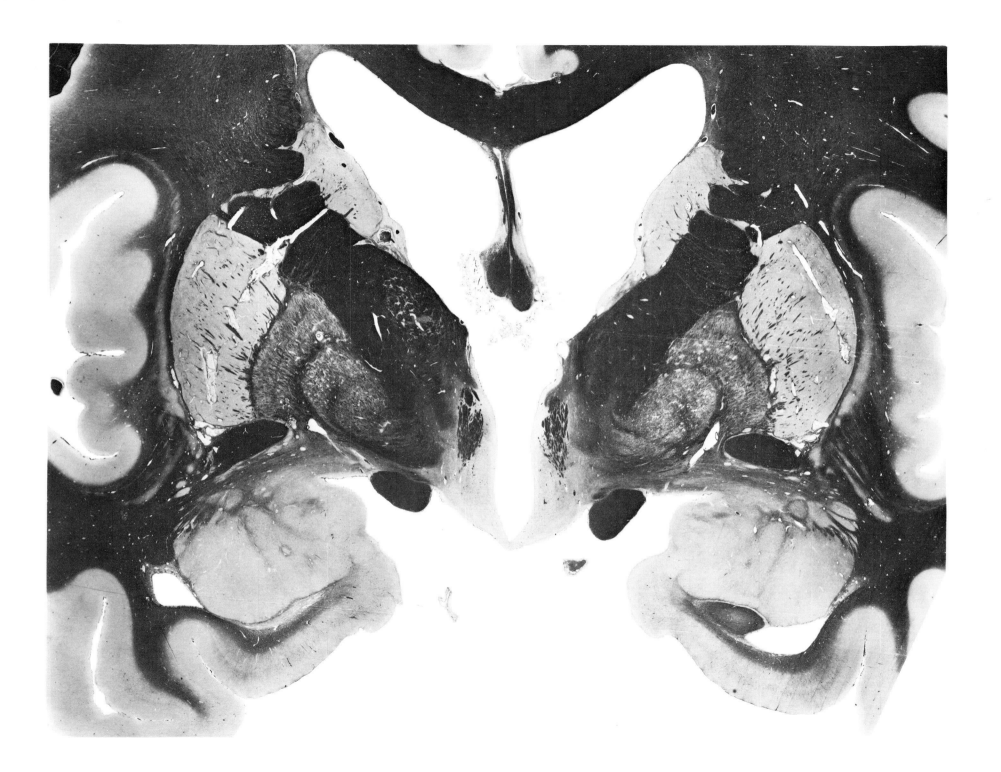

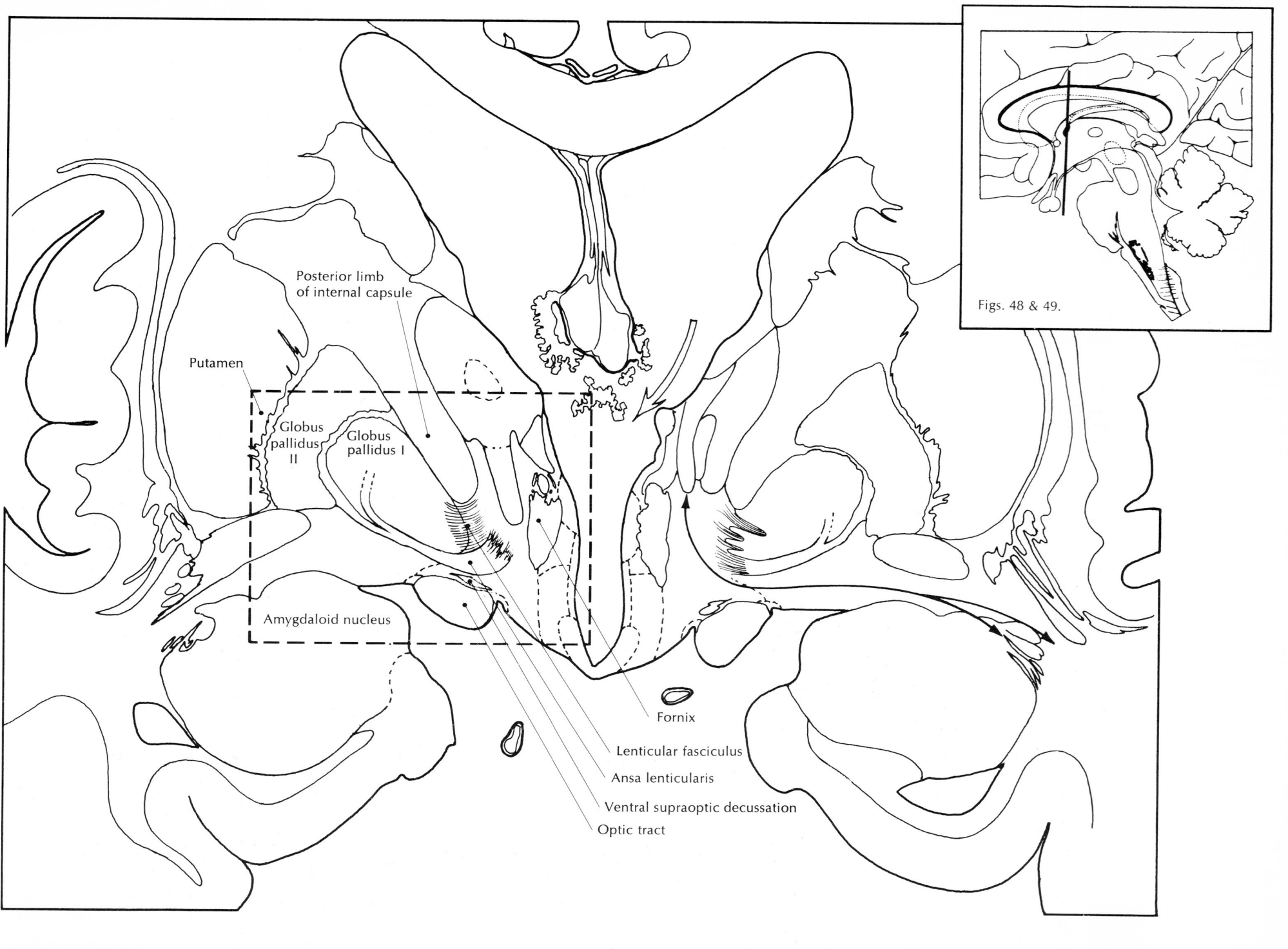

Posterior limb
of internal capsule

Putamen

Globus
pallidus
II

Globus
pallidus I

Amygdaloid nucleus

Figs. 48 & 49.

Fornix

Lenticular fasciculus

Ansa lenticularis

Ventral supraoptic decussation

Optic tract

Figure 49. Detail of ansa lenticularis and lenticular fasciculus emerging from globus pallidus—Weil, 12X

98

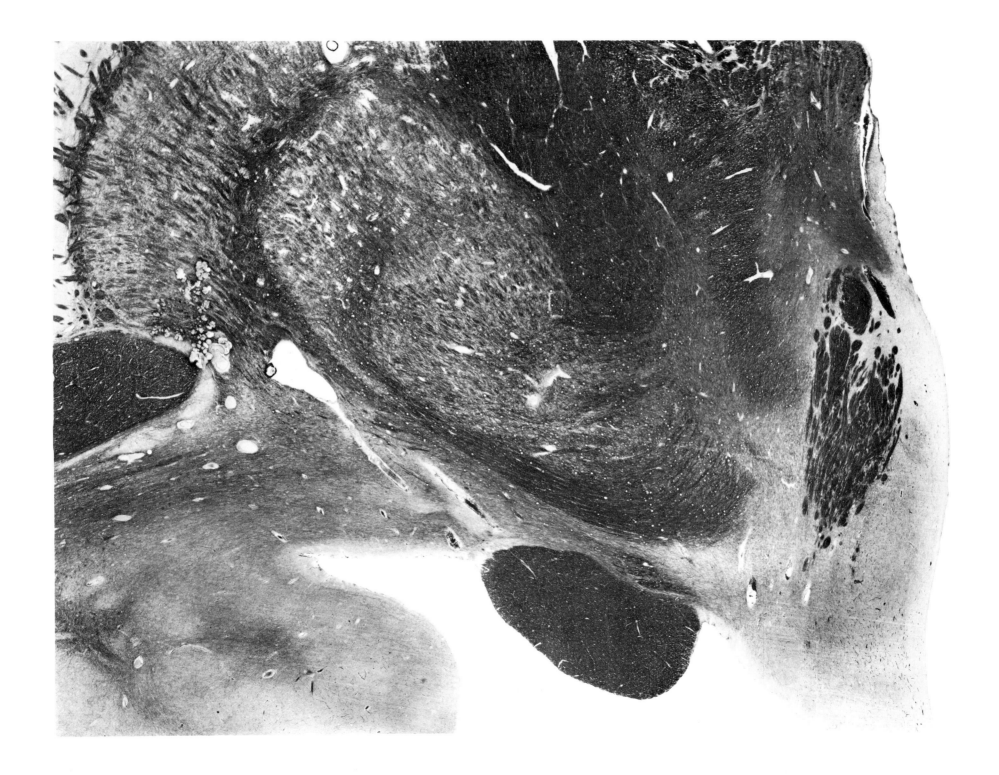

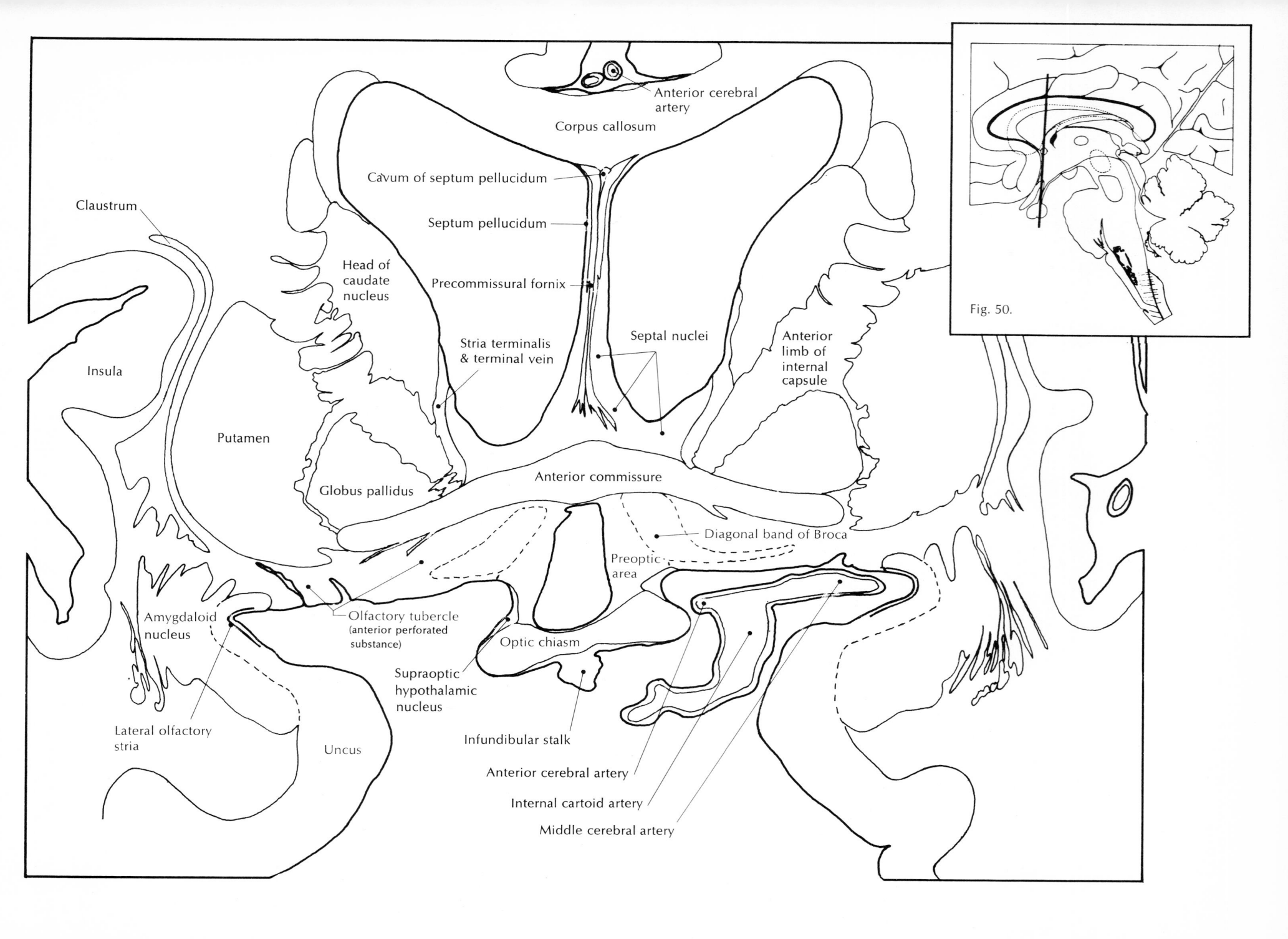

Claustrum

Insula

Head of
caudate
nucleus

Putamen

Globus pallidus

Amygdaloid
nucleus

Lateral olfactory
stria

Uncus

Anterior cerebral
artery

Corpus callosum

Cavum of septum pellucidum

Septum pellucidum

Precommissural fornix

Septal nuclei

Anterior
limb of
internal
capsule

Stria terminalis
& terminal vein

Anterior commissure

Diagonal band of Broca

Preoptic
area

Olfactory tubercle
(anterior perforated
substance)

Optic chiasm

Supraoptic
hypothalamic
nucleus

Infundibular stalk

Anterior cerebral artery

Internal cartoid artery

Middle cerebral artery

Fig. 50.

Figure 50. Basal ganglia at the level of the anterior commissure—Weil, 4X

100

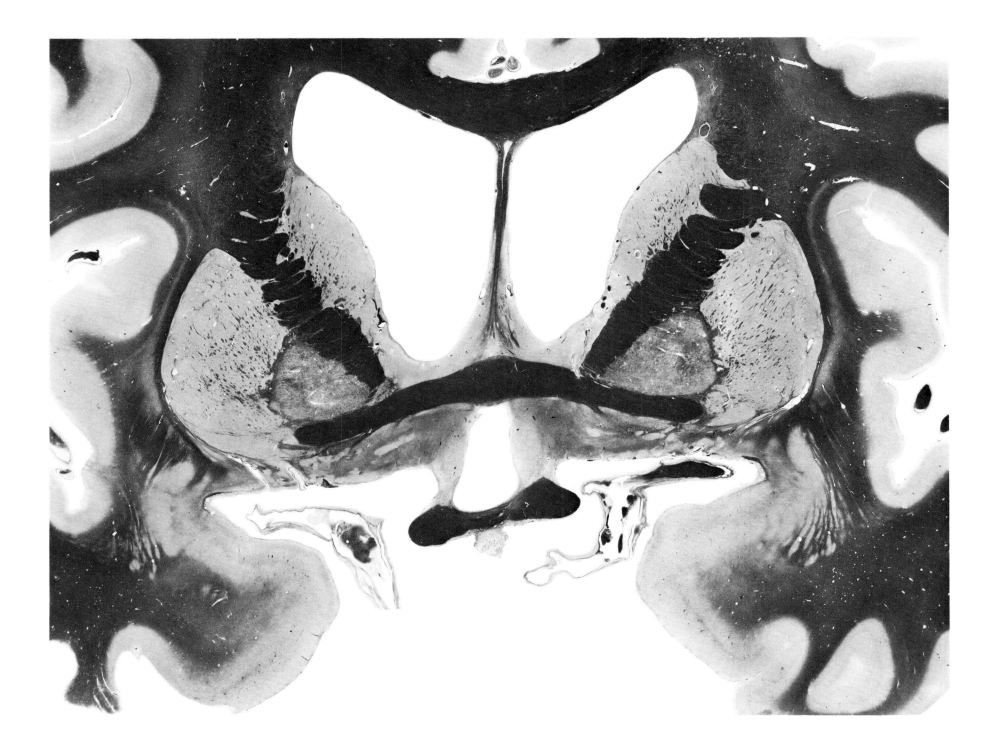

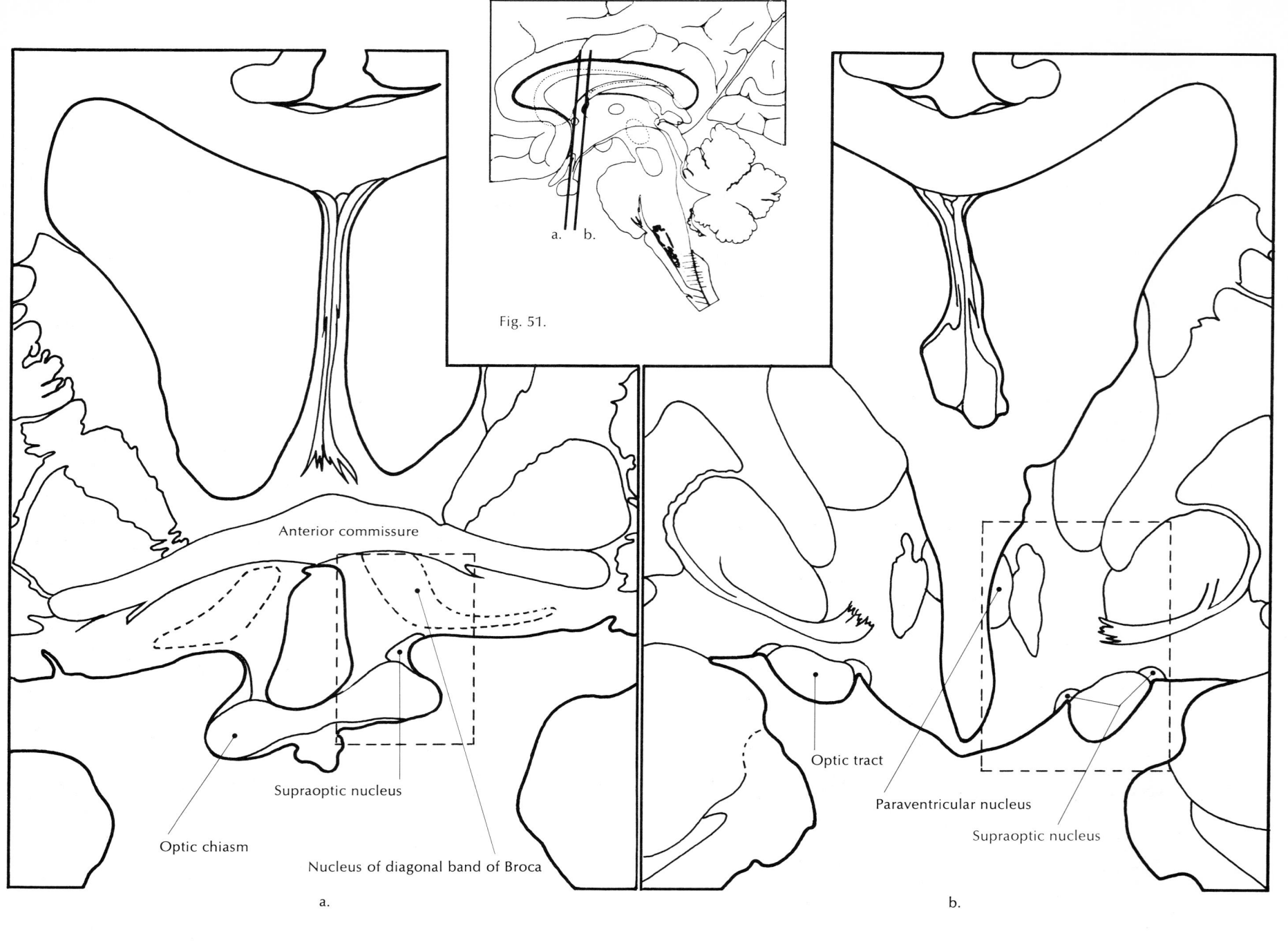

Fig. 51.

Anterior commissure

Supraoptic nucleus

Optic chiasm

Nucleus of diagonal band of Broca

a.

Optic tract

Paraventricular nucleus

Supraoptic nucleus

b.

Figure 51. The paraventricular and supraoptic hypothalamic nuclei. a. Section at the level of the anterior commissure—Nissl, 16X b. Section caudal to the anterior commissure through the tuberal region of the hypothalamus—Nissl, 16X

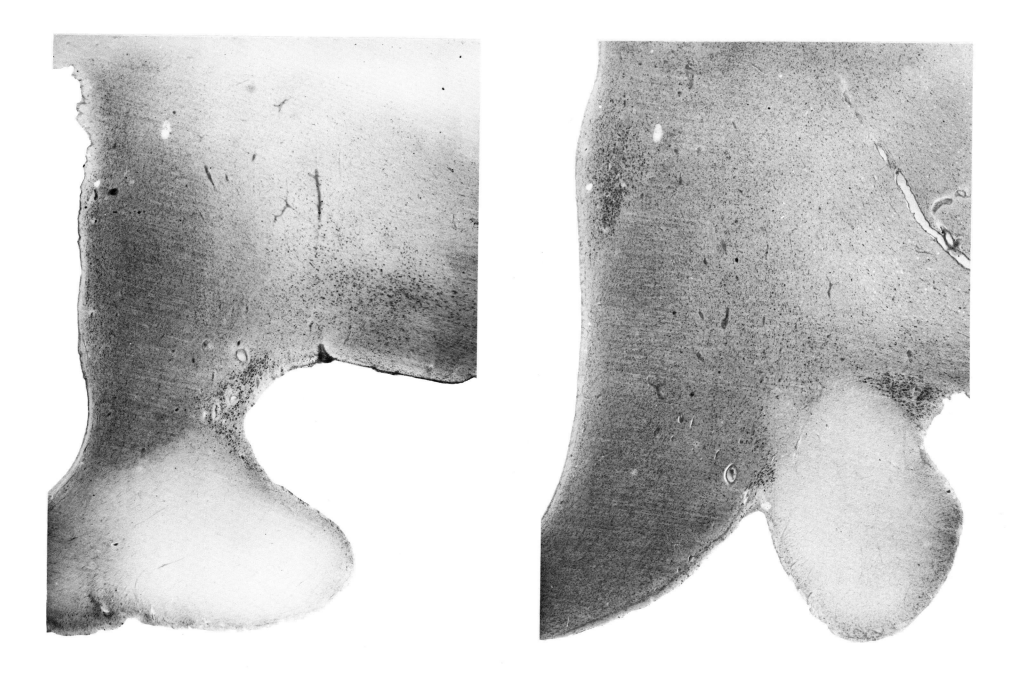

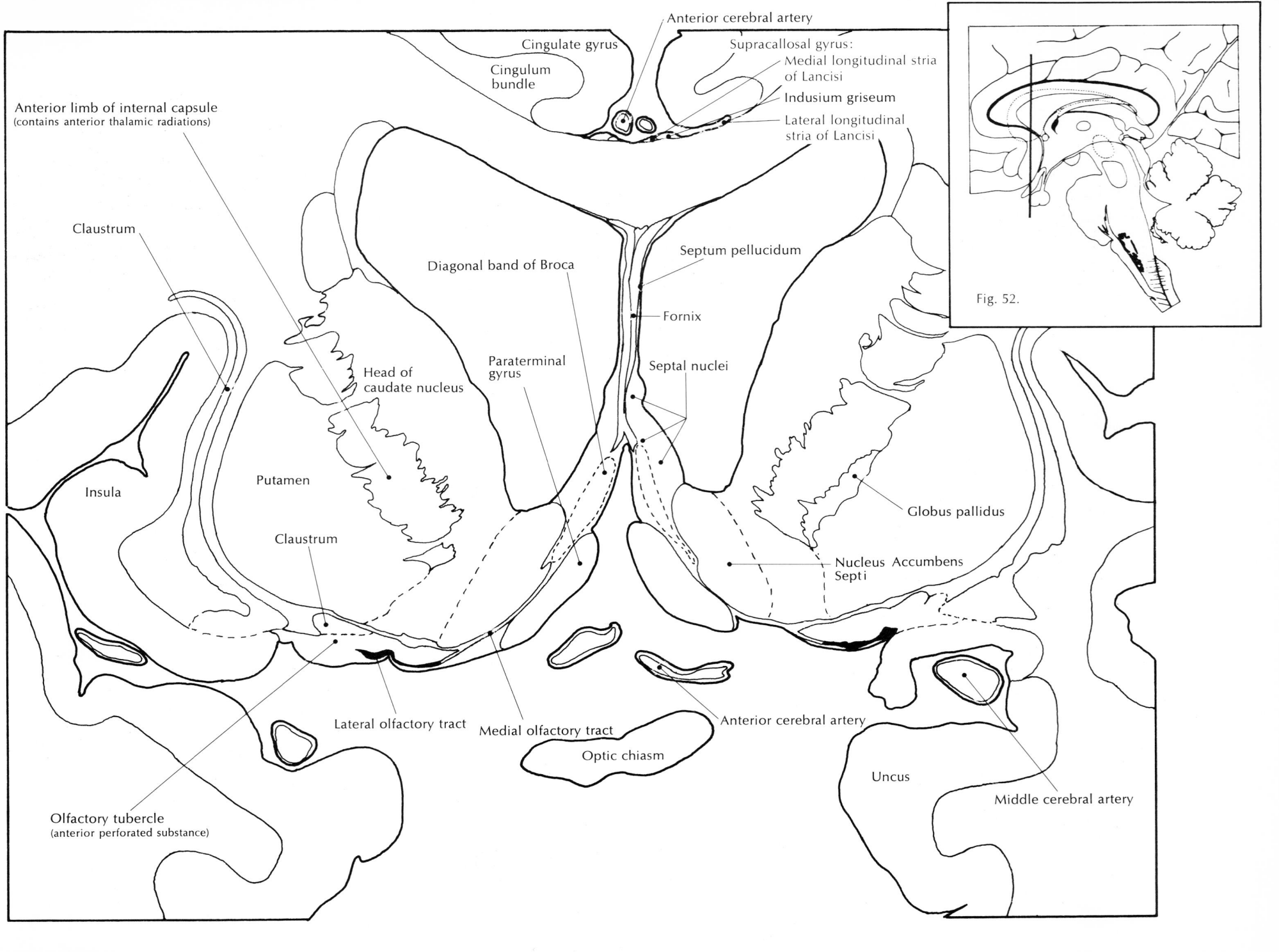

Figure 52. Basal ganglia rostral to anterior commissure, head of the caudate nucleus— Weil, 4X

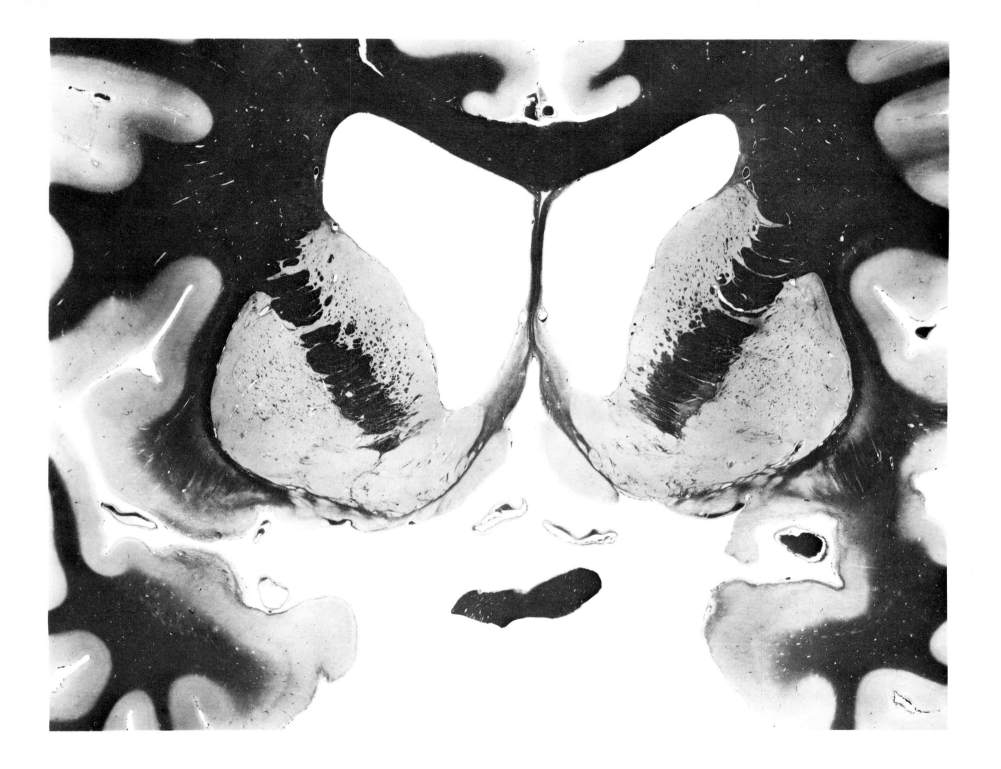

SAGITTAL SECTIONS OF THE BRAIN STEM, DIENCEPHALON, AND BASAL GANGLIA

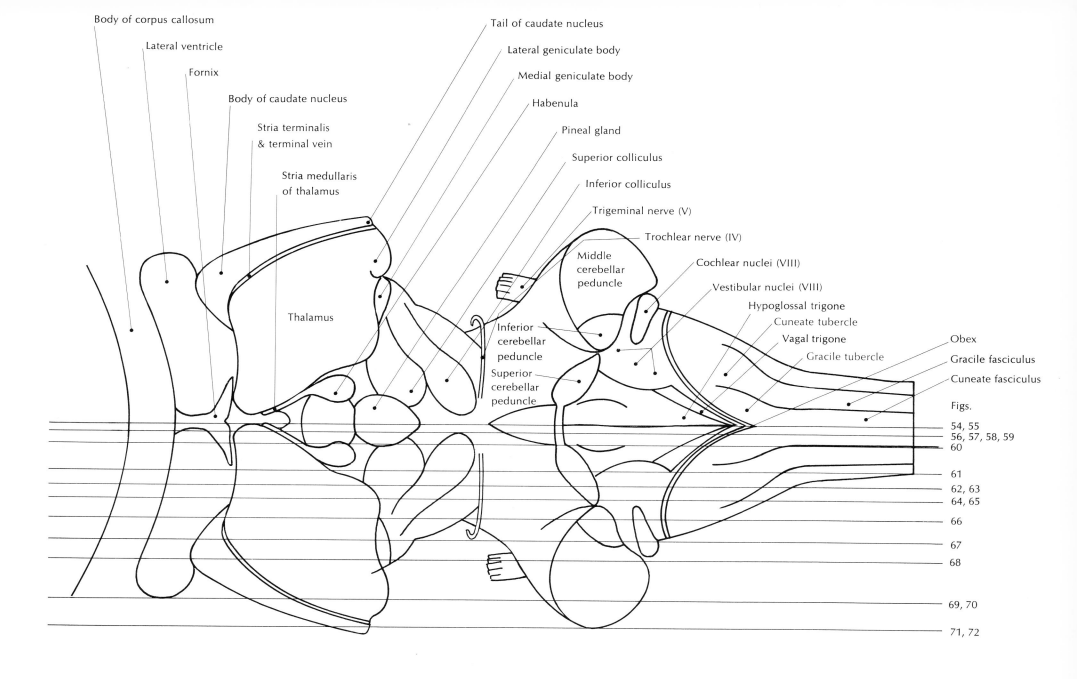

Body of corpus callosum

Lateral ventricle

Fornix

Body of caudate nucleus

Stria terminalis
& terminal vein

Stria medullaris
of thalamus

Tail of caudate nucleus

Lateral geniculate body

Medial geniculate body

Habenula

Pineal gland

Superior colliculus

Inferior colliculus

Trigeminal nerve (V)

Trochlear nerve (IV)

Cochlear nuclei (VIII)

Vestibular nuclei (VIII)

Hypoglossal trigone

Cuneate tubercle

Vagal trigone

Gracile tubercle

Obex

Gracile fasciculus

Cuneate fasciculus

Middle
cerebellar
peduncle

Inferior
cerebellar
peduncle

Superior
cerebellar
peduncle

Thalamus

Figs.

54, 55
56, 57, 58, 59
60

61

62, 63
64, 65

66

67

68

69, 70

71, 72

Figure 53. Dorsal surface of the brain stem and diencephalon indicating the locations
of the sagittal sections of the brain stem, diencephalon, and basal ganglia

107

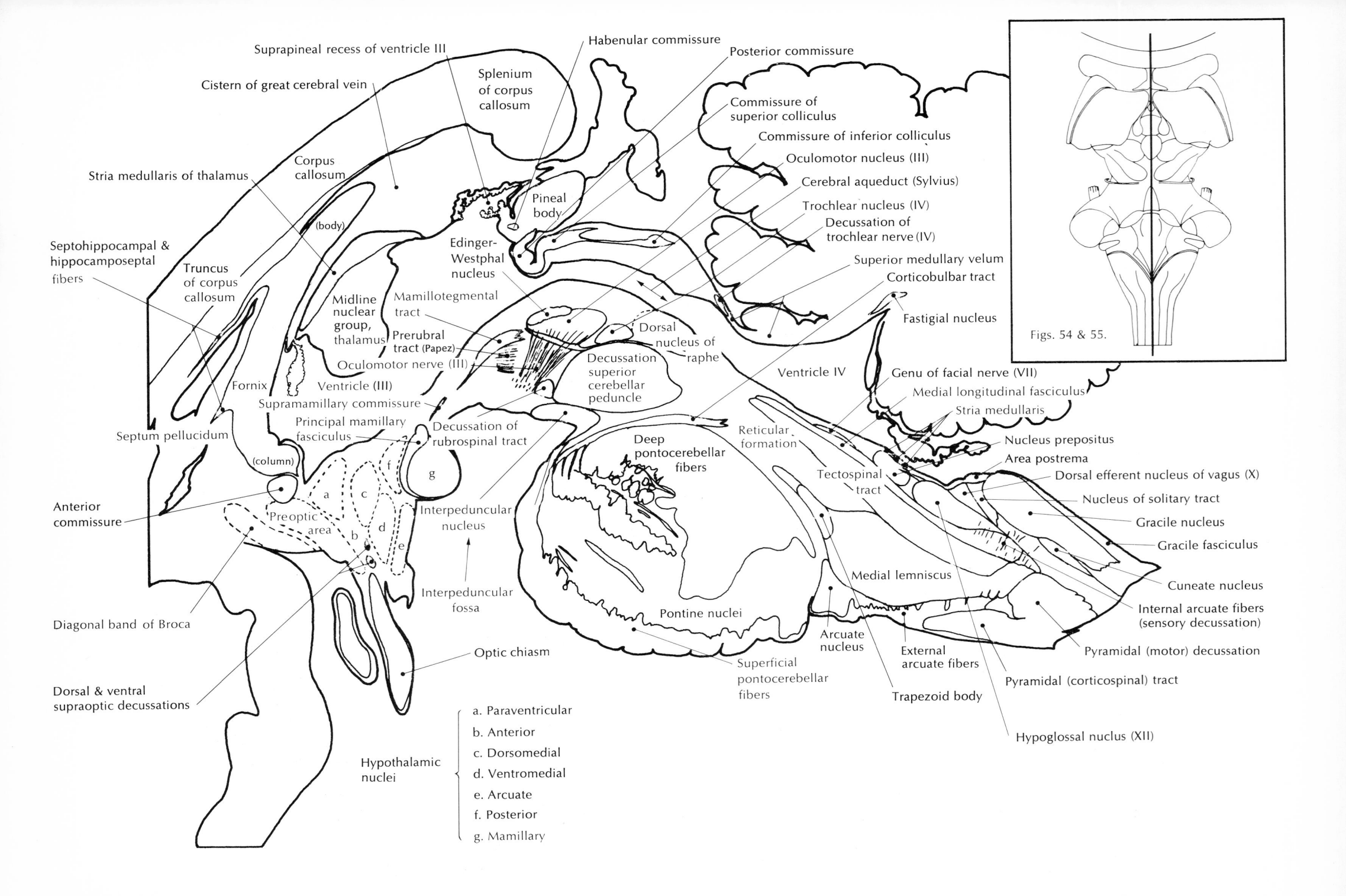

Suprapineal recess of ventricle III

Cistern of great cerebral vein

Stria medullaris of thalamus

Corpus callosum (body)

Septohippocampal & hippocamposeptal fibers

Truncus of corpus callosum

Midline nuclear group, thalamus

Mamillotegmental tract

Prerubral tract (Papez)

Oculomotor nerve (III)

Fornix

Ventricle (III)

Supramamillary commissure

Principal mamillary fasciculus

Septum pellucidum

(column)

Anterior commissure

Diagonal band of Broca

Dorsal & ventral supraoptic decussations

Edinger-Westphal nucleus

Decussation of rubrospinal tract

Preoptic area

Interpeduncular nucleus

Interpeduncular fossa

Optic chiasm

Habenular commissure

Splenium of corpus callosum

Pineal body

Posterior commissure

Commissure of superior colliculus

Commissure of inferior colliculus

Oculomotor nucleus (III)

Cerebral aqueduct (Sylvius)

Trochlear nucleus (IV)

Decussation of trochlear nerve (IV)

Superior medullary velum

Corticobulbar tract

Fastigial nucleus

Figs. 54 & 55.

Dorsal nucleus of raphe

Decussation superior cerebellar peduncle

Deep pontocerebellar fibers

Reticular formation

Ventricle IV

Genu of facial nerve (VII)

Medial longitudinal fasciculus

Stria medullaris

Tectospinal tract

Nucleus prepositus

Area postrema

Dorsal efferent nucleus of vagus (X)

Nucleus of solitary tract

Gracile nucleus

Gracile fasciculus

Cuneate nucleus

Internal arcuate fibers (sensory decussation)

Pyramidal (motor) decussation

Pyramidal (corticospinal) tract

Hypoglossal nucleus (XII)

Medial lemniscus

Pontine nuclei

Arcuate nucleus

External arcuate fibers

Trapezoid body

Superficial pontocerebellar fibers

Hypothalamic nuclei
a. Paraventricular
b. Anterior
c. Dorsomedial
d. Ventromedial
e. Arcuate
f. Posterior
g. Mamillary

Figure 54. Midsagittal section—Weil, 3.5X

108

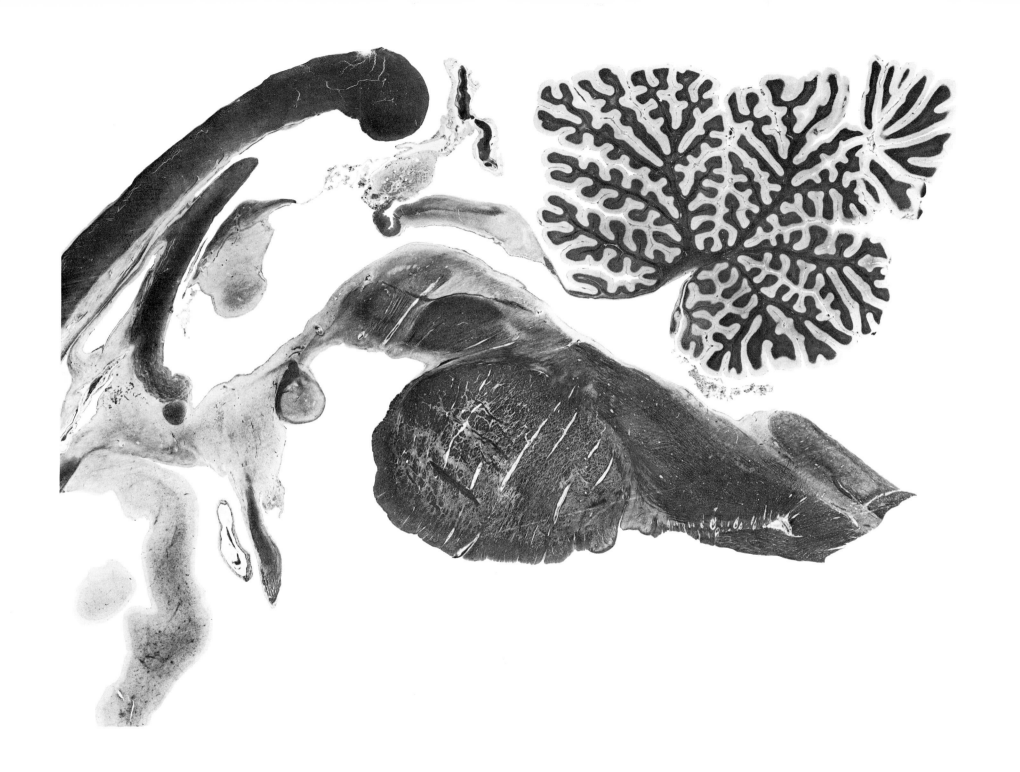

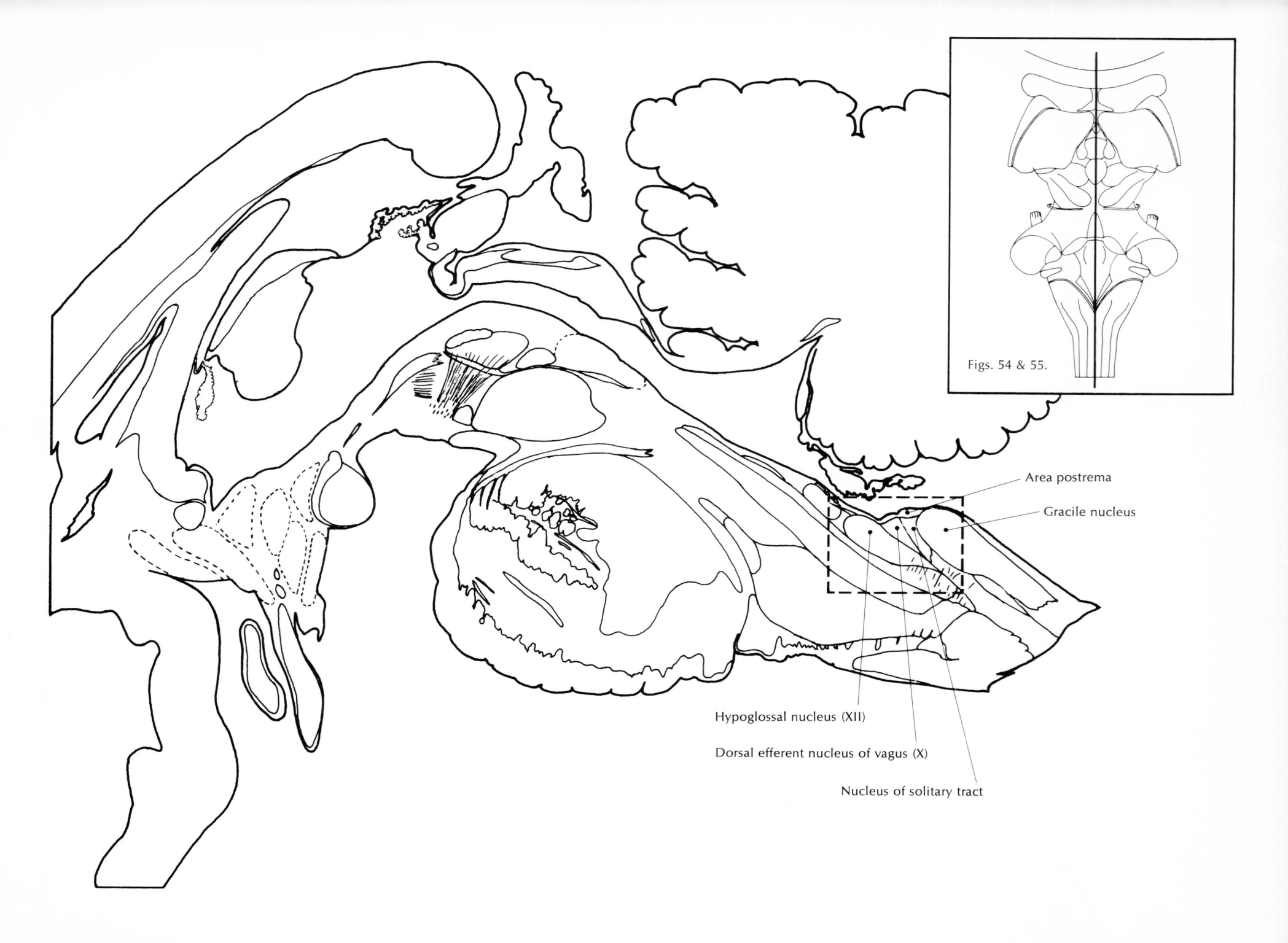

Area postrema

Gracile nucleus

Hypoglossal nucleus (XII)

Dorsal efferent nucleus of vagus (X)

Nucleus of solitary tract

Figs. 54 & 55.

Figure 55. Detail of the hypoglossal nucleus—Nissl, 38X

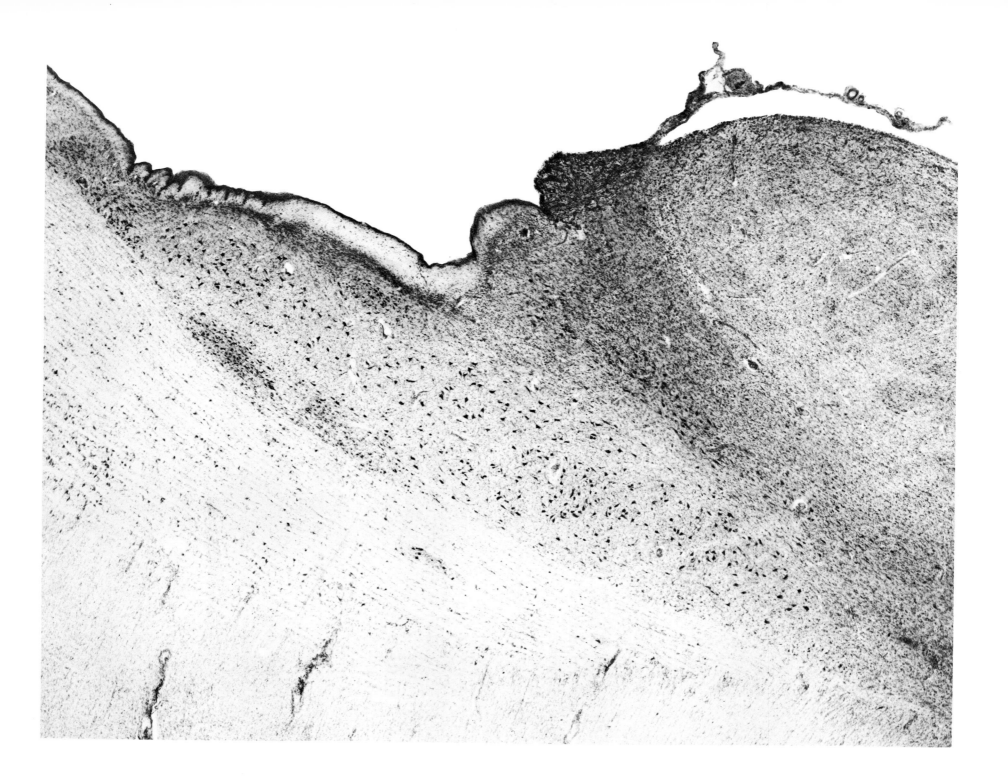

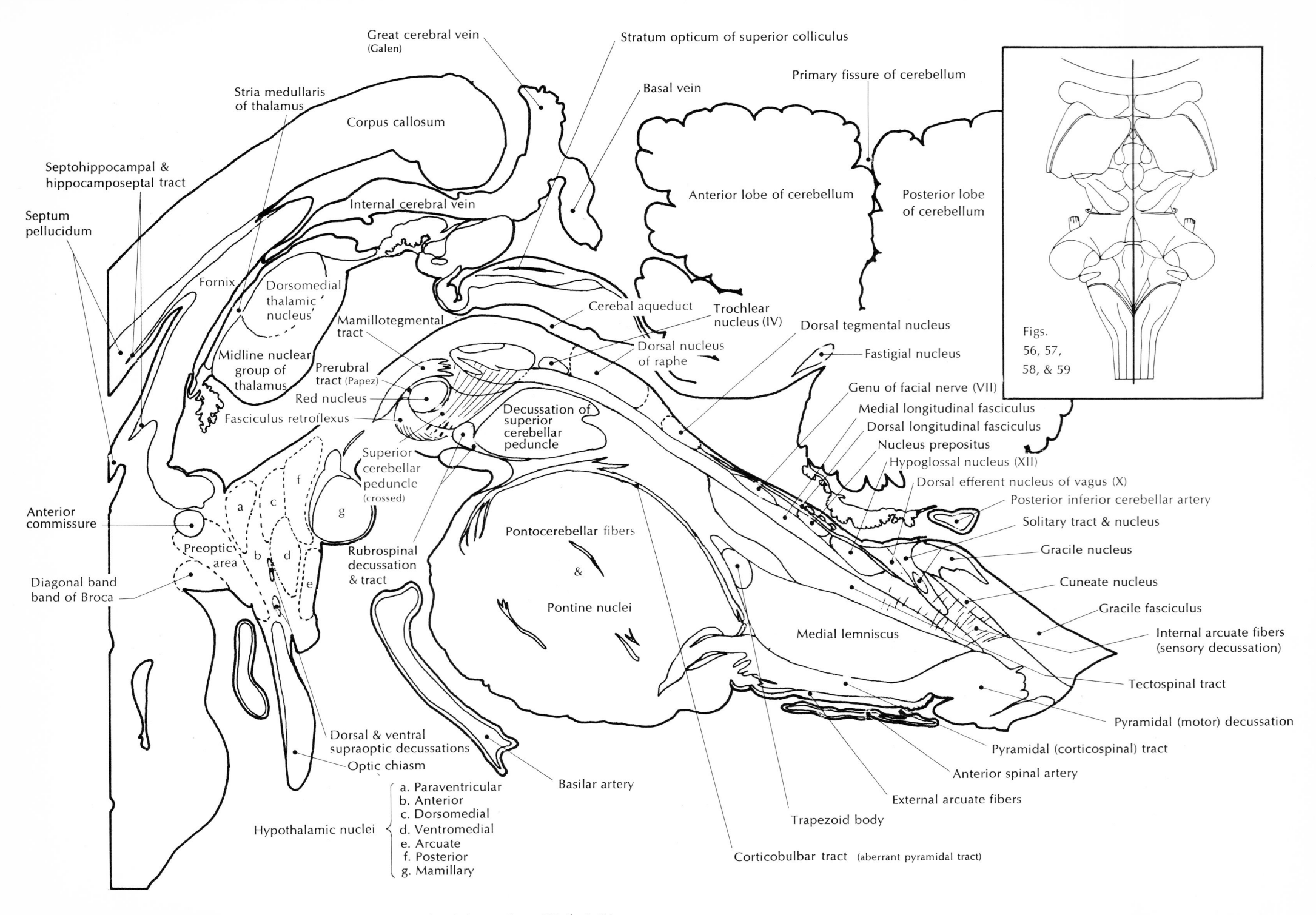

Figure 56. Parasagittal section through the medial longitudinal fasciculus—Weil, 3.5X

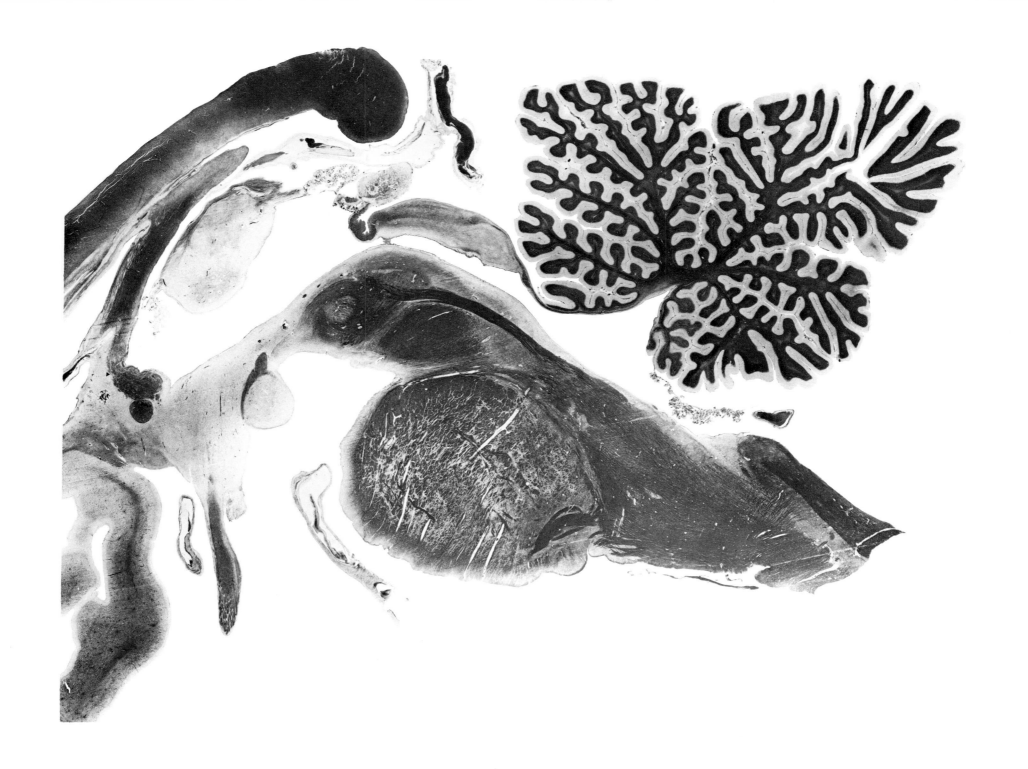

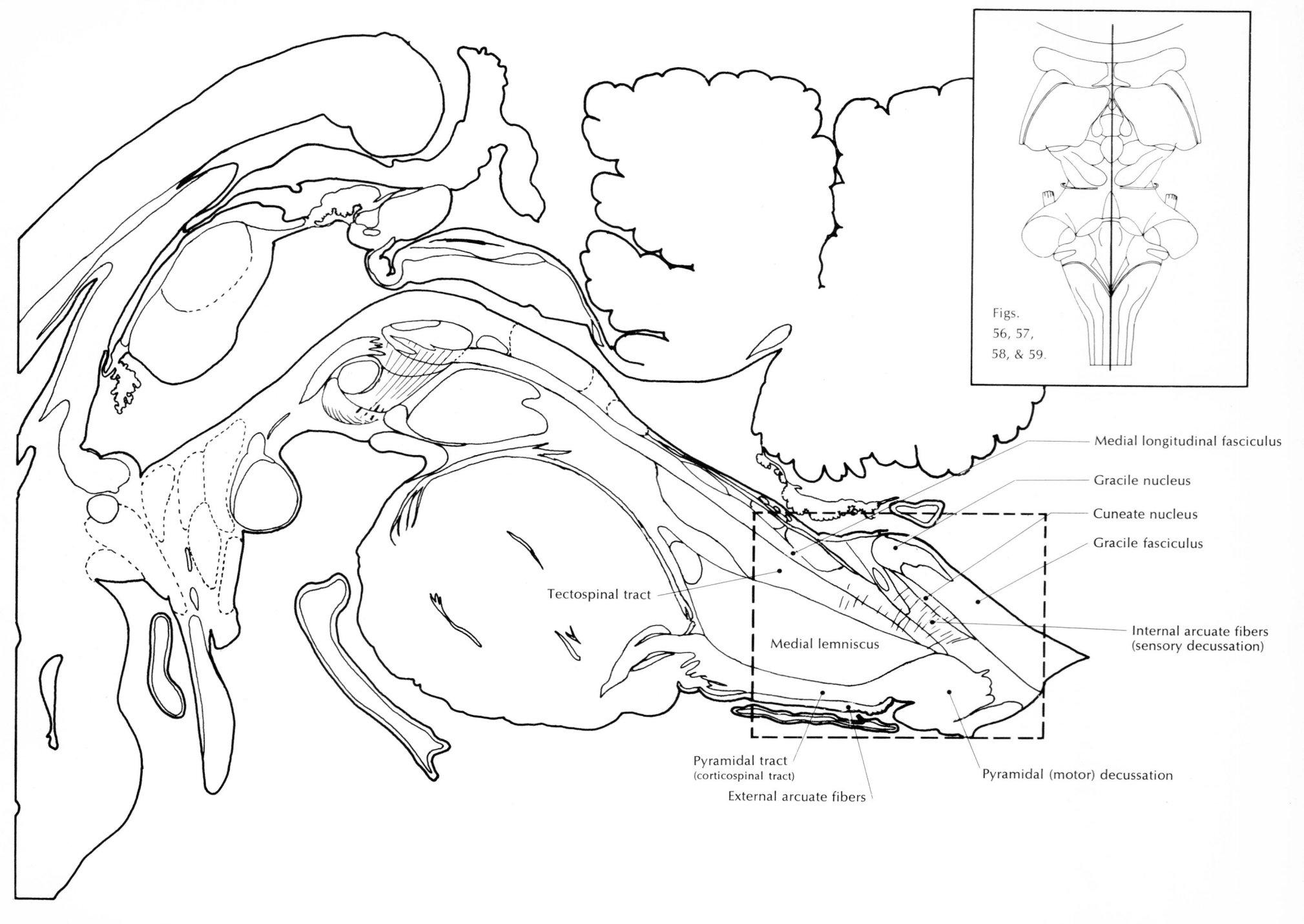

Medial longitudinal fasciculus

Gracile nucleus

Cuneate nucleus

Gracile fasciculus

Internal arcuate fibers
(sensory decussation)

Tectospinal tract

Medial lemniscus

Figs.
56, 57,
58, & 59.

Pyramidal tract
(corticospinal tract)

External arcuate fibers

Pyramidal (motor) decussation

Figure 57. Detail of the motor and sensory decussations in the caudal half of the medulla—Weil, 14X

114

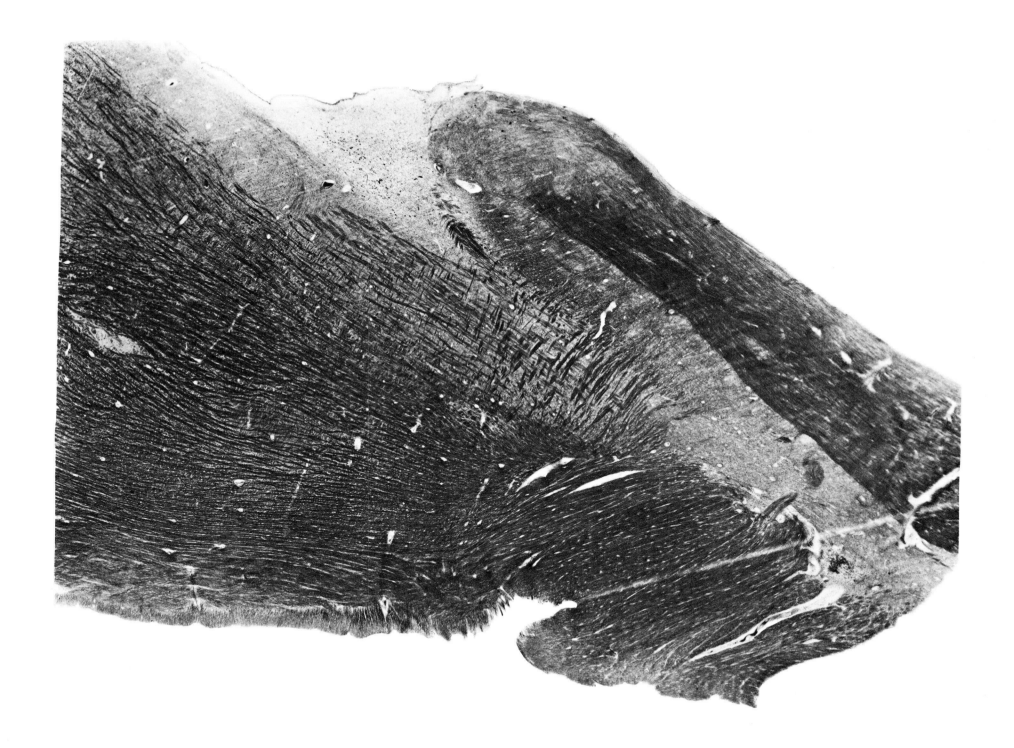

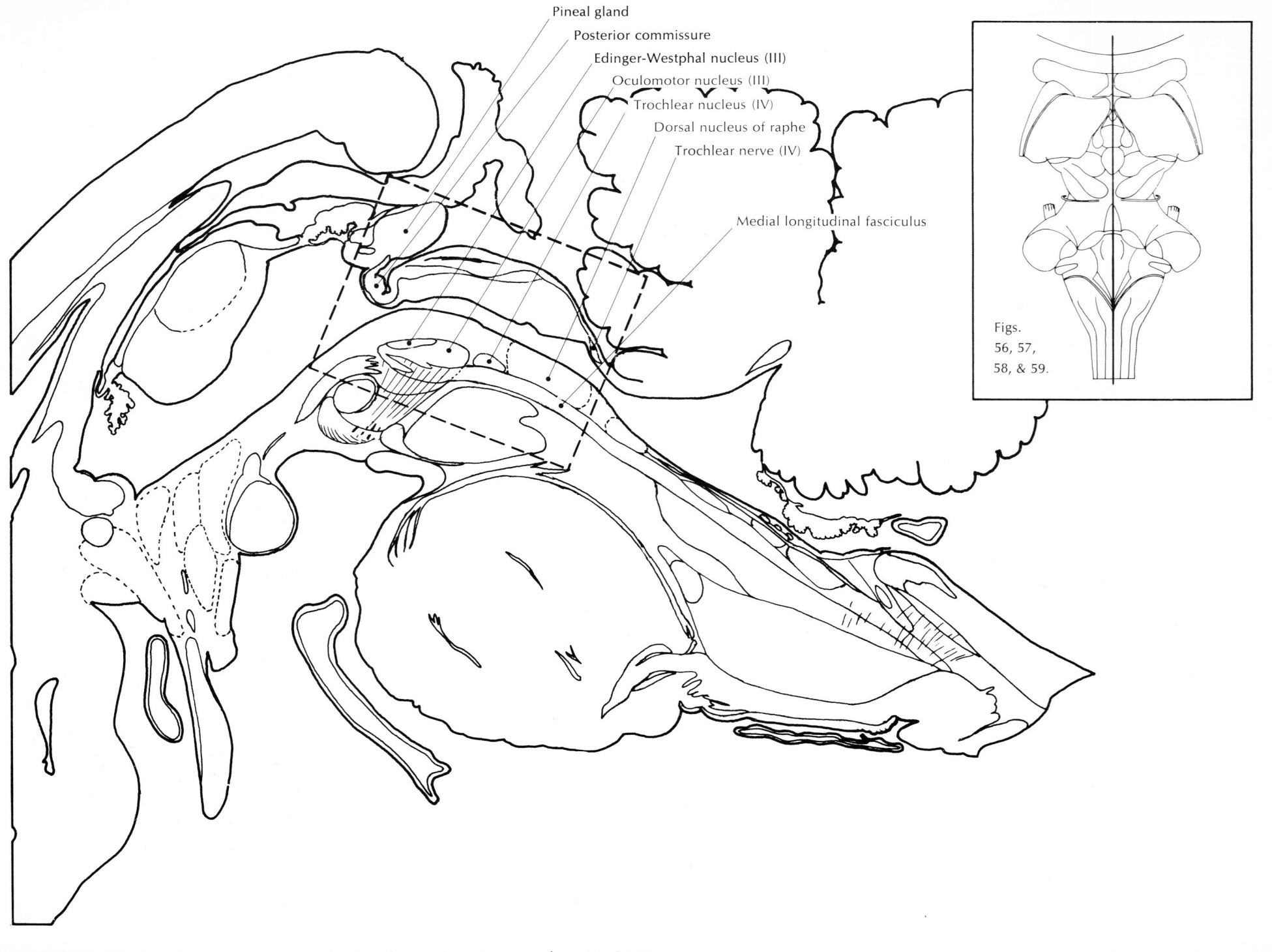

Pineal gland
Posterior commissure
Edinger-Westphal nucleus (III)
Oculomotor nucleus (III)
Trochlear nucleus (IV)
Dorsal nucleus of raphe
Trochlear nerve (IV)

Medial longitudinal fasciculus

Figs.
56, 57,
58, & 59.

Figure 58. Detail of periaqueductal gray region of midbrain—the oculomotor complex—Nissl, 15X

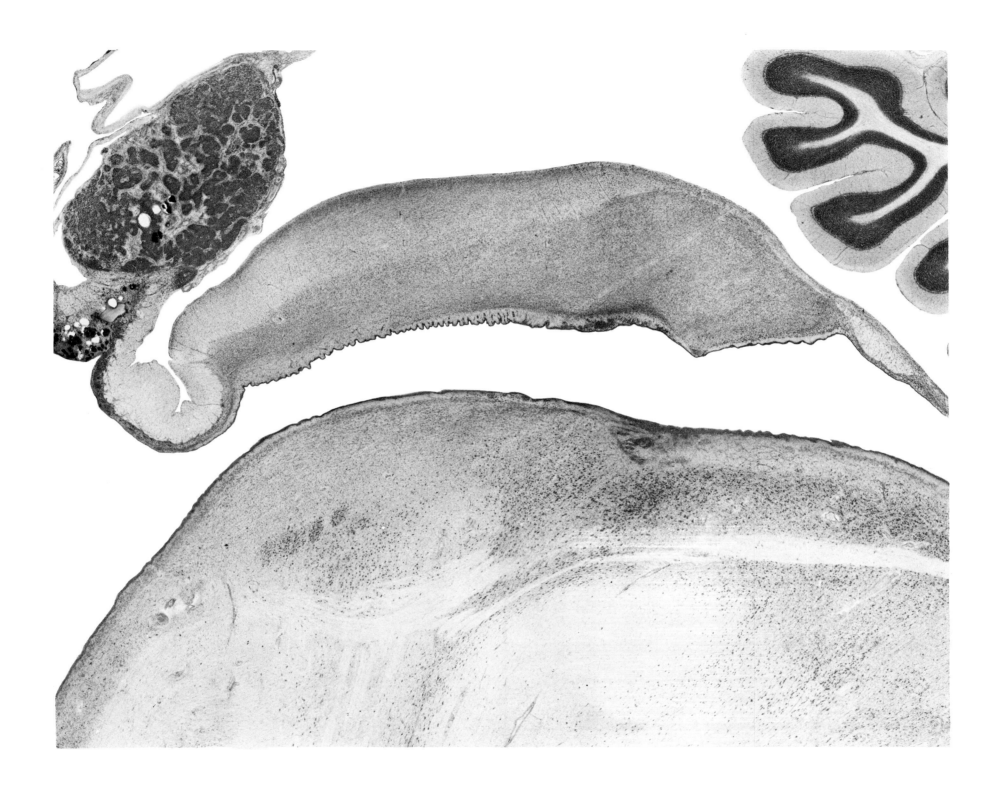

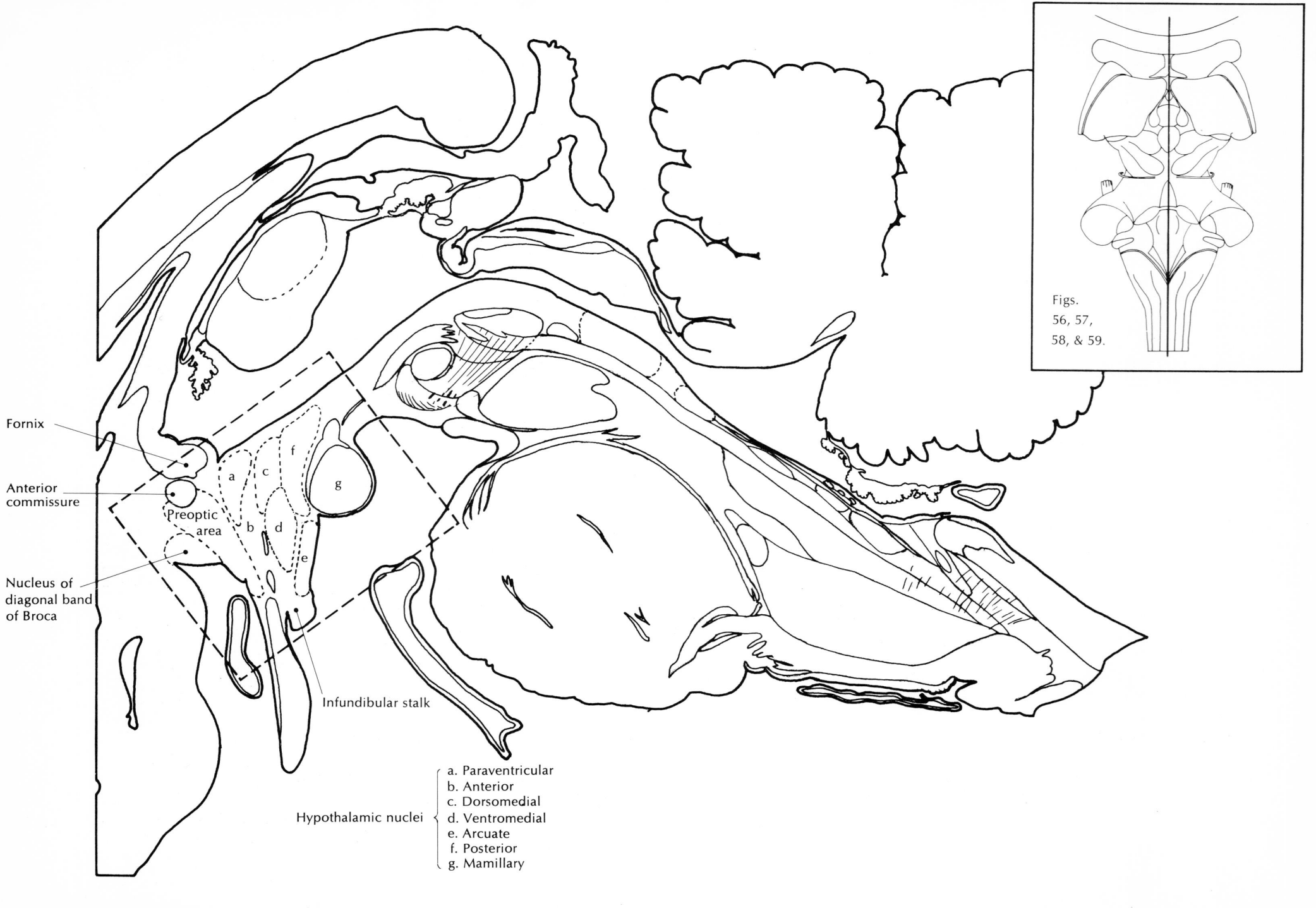

Fornix

Anterior commissure

Preoptic area

Nucleus of diagonal band of Broca

Infundibular stalk

Figs. 56, 57, 58, & 59.

Hypothalamic nuclei {
a. Paraventricular
b. Anterior
c. Dorsomedial
d. Ventromedial
e. Arcuate
f. Posterior
g. Mamillary
}

Figure 59. Hypothalamic nuclei (the paraventricular nucleus is the only one easily seen in the photograph)—Nissl, 15X

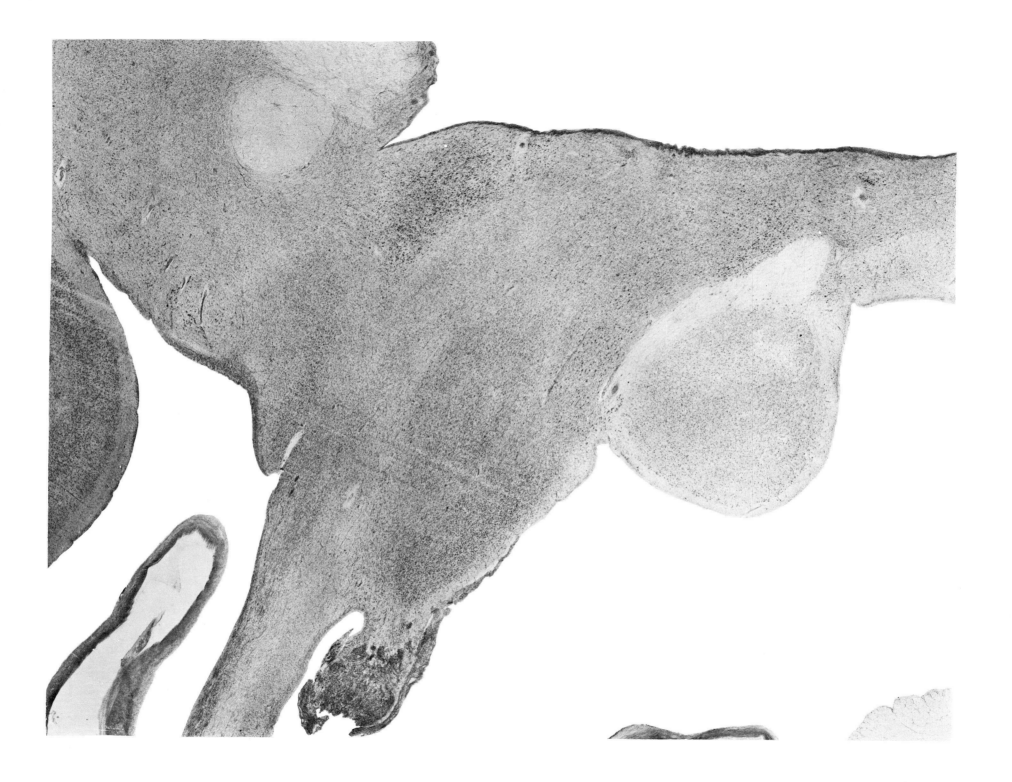

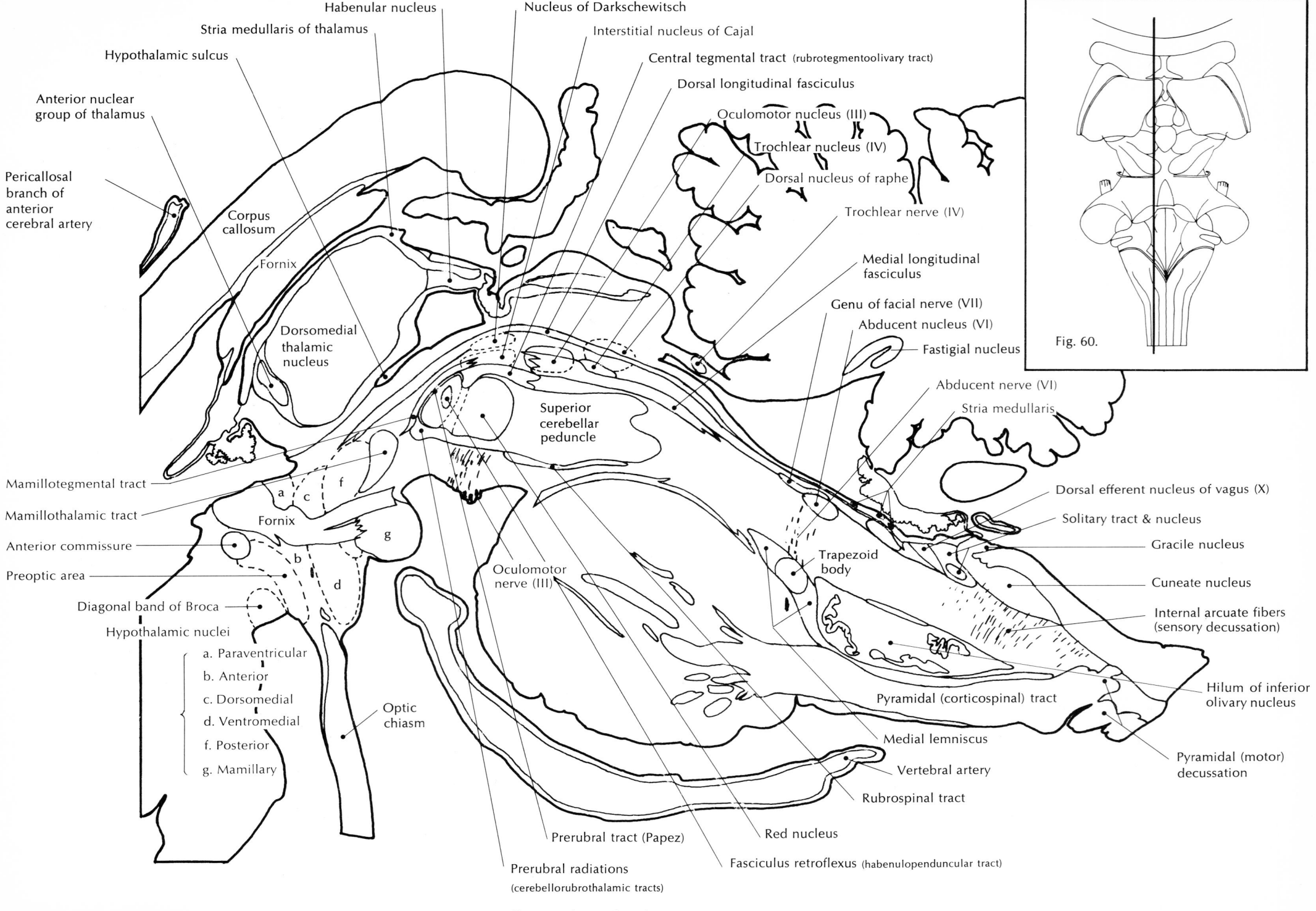

Anterior nuclear group of thalamus

Pericallosal branch of anterior cerebral artery

Hypothalamic sulcus

Stria medullaris of thalamus

Habenular nucleus

Nucleus of Darkschewitsch

Interstitial nucleus of Cajal

Central tegmental tract (rubrotegmentoolivary tract)

Dorsal longitudinal fasciculus

Oculomotor nucleus (III)

Trochlear nucleus (IV)

Dorsal nucleus of raphe

Trochlear nerve (IV)

Medial longitudinal fasciculus

Genu of facial nerve (VII)

Abducent nucleus (VI)

Fastigial nucleus

Abducent nerve (VI)

Stria medullaris

Fig. 60.

Corpus callosum

Fornix

Dorsomedial thalamic nucleus

Superior cerebellar peduncle

Mamillotegmental tract

Mamillothalamic tract

Anterior commissure

Preoptic area

Diagonal band of Broca

Hypothalamic nuclei

a. Paraventricular
b. Anterior
c. Dorsomedial
d. Ventromedial
f. Posterior
g. Mamillary

Fornix

a c f

b

d

g

Optic chiasm

Oculomotor nerve (III)

Trapezoid body

Dorsal efferent nucleus of vagus (X)

Solitary tract & nucleus

Gracile nucleus

Cuneate nucleus

Internal arcuate fibers (sensory decussation)

Hilum of inferior olivary nucleus

Pyramidal (corticospinal) tract

Medial lemniscus

Pyramidal (motor) decussation

Vertebral artery

Rubrospinal tract

Red nucleus

Prerubral tract (Papez)

Fasciculus retroflexus (habenulopenduncular tract)

Prerubral radiations

(cerebellorubrothalamic tracts)

Figure 60. Parasagittal section through the fornix terminating in the mamillary nucleus —Weil, 3.5X

120

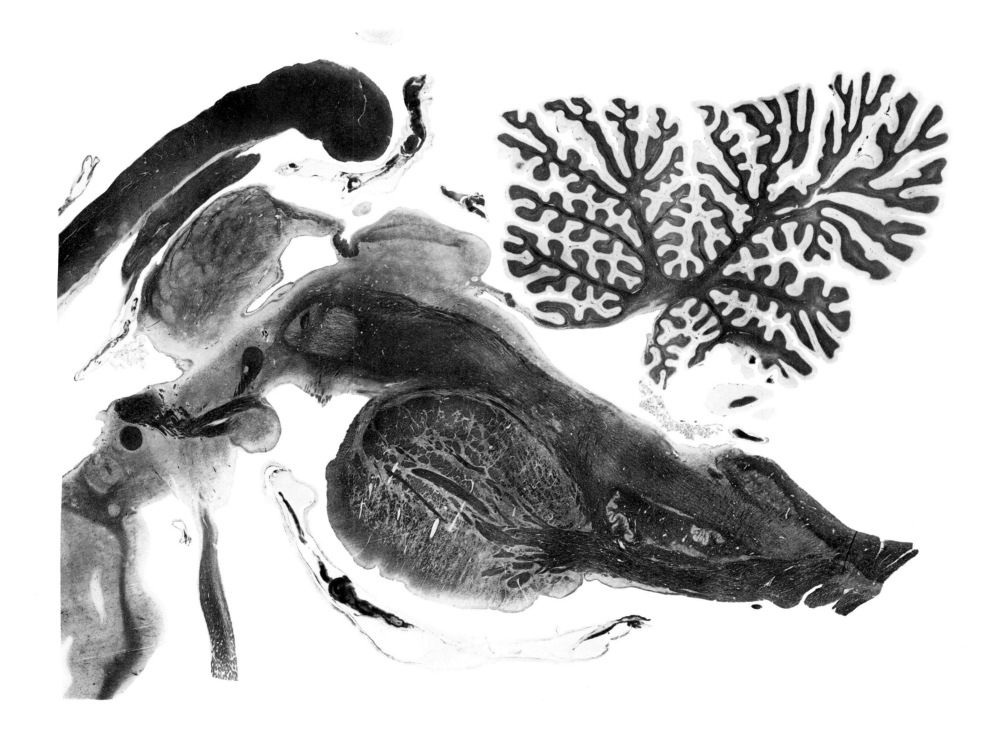

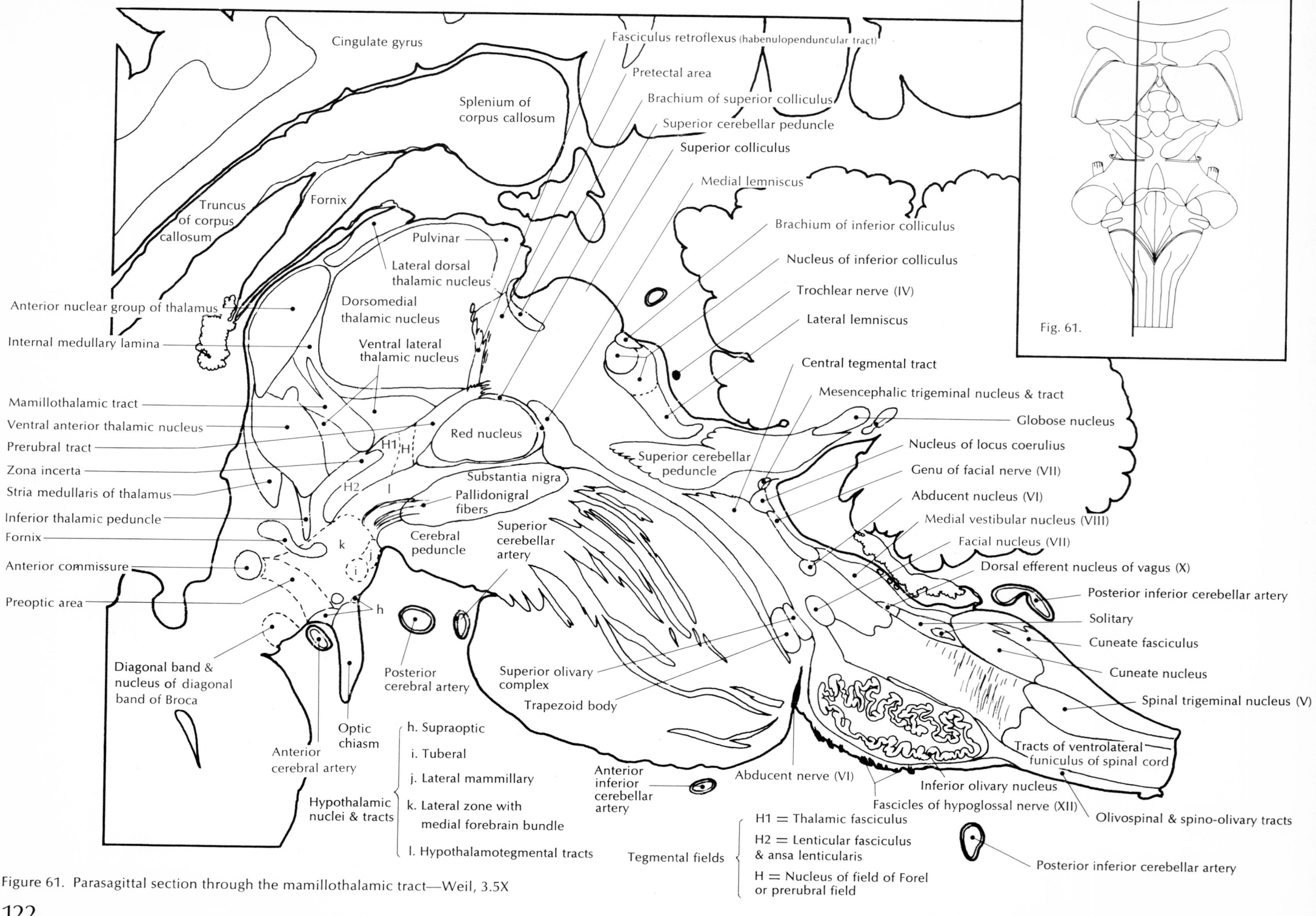

Cingulate gyrus

Fasciculus retroflexus (habenulopenduncular tract)

Pretectal area

Brachium of superior colliculus

Splenium of corpus callosum

Superior cerebellar peduncle

Superior colliculus

Medial lemniscus

Truncus of corpus callosum

Fornix

Brachium of inferior colliculus

Nucleus of inferior colliculus

Pulvinar

Lateral dorsal thalamic nucleus

Trochlear nerve (IV)

Anterior nuclear group of thalamus

Dorsomedial thalamic nucleus

Lateral lemniscus

Internal medullary lamina

Ventral lateral thalamic nucleus

Central tegmental tract

Mesencephalic trigeminal nucleus & tract

Red nucleus

Globose nucleus

Mamillothalamic tract

Superior cerebellar peduncle

Nucleus of locus coerulius

Ventral anterior thalamic nucleus

H1 H

Genu of facial nerve (VII)

Prerubral tract

Substantia nigra

Abducent nucleus (VI)

Zona incerta

H2 l

Pallidonigral fibers

Medial vestibular nucleus (VIII)

Stria medullaris of thalamus

Superior cerebellar artery

Facial nucleus (VII)

Inferior thalamic peduncle

Cerebral peduncle

Superior cerebellar

Dorsal efferent nucleus of vagus (X)

Fornix

k

j

Posterior inferior cerebellar artery

Anterior commissure

i

Solitary

Preoptic area

h

Cuneate fasciculus

Diagonal band & nucleus of diagonal band of Broca

Cuneate nucleus

Posterior cerebral artery

Superior olivary complex

Spinal trigeminal nucleus (V)

Optic chiasm

Trapezoid body

Anterior cerebral artery

h. Supraoptic

Tracts of ventrolateral funiculus of spinal cord

Anterior inferior cerebellar artery

i. Tuberal

Abducent nerve (VI)

Inferior olivary nucleus

j. Lateral mammillary

k. Lateral zone with medial forebrain bundle

Fascicles of hypoglossal nerve (XII)

Olivospinal & spino-olivary tracts

Hypothalamic nuclei & tracts

H1 = Thalamic fasciculus

l. Hypothalamotegmental tracts

Tegmental fields

H2 = Lenticular fasciculus & ansa lenticularis

Posterior inferior cerebellar artery

H = Nucleus of field of Forel or prerubral field

Fig. 61.

Figure 61. Parasagittal section through the mamillothalamic tract—Weil, 3.5X

122

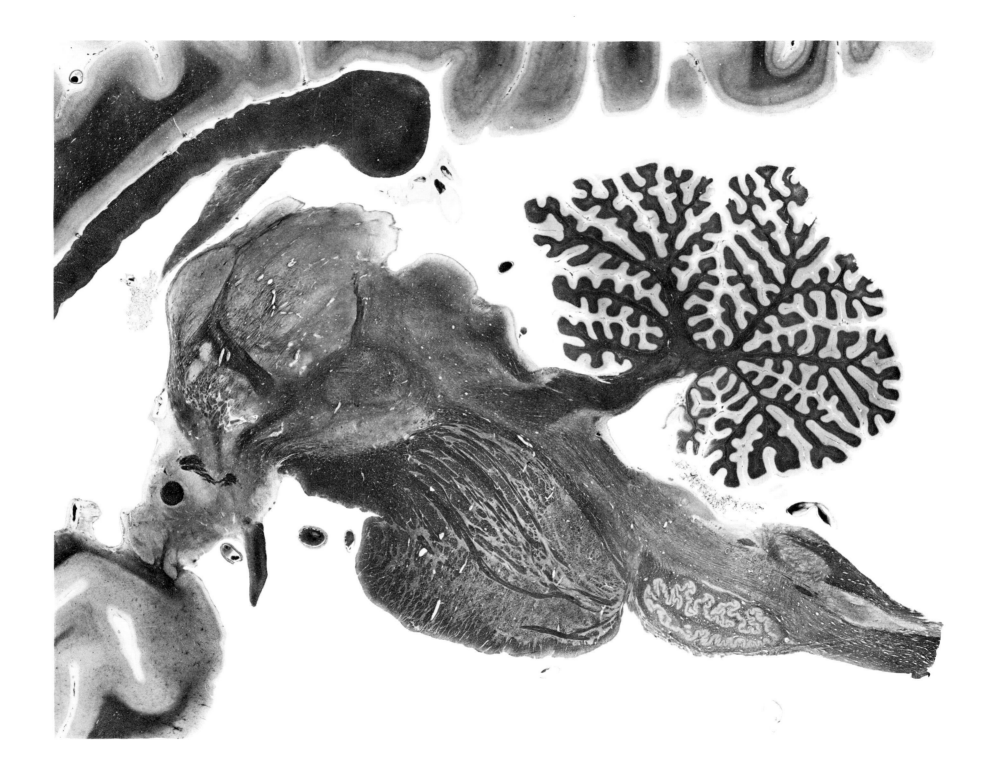

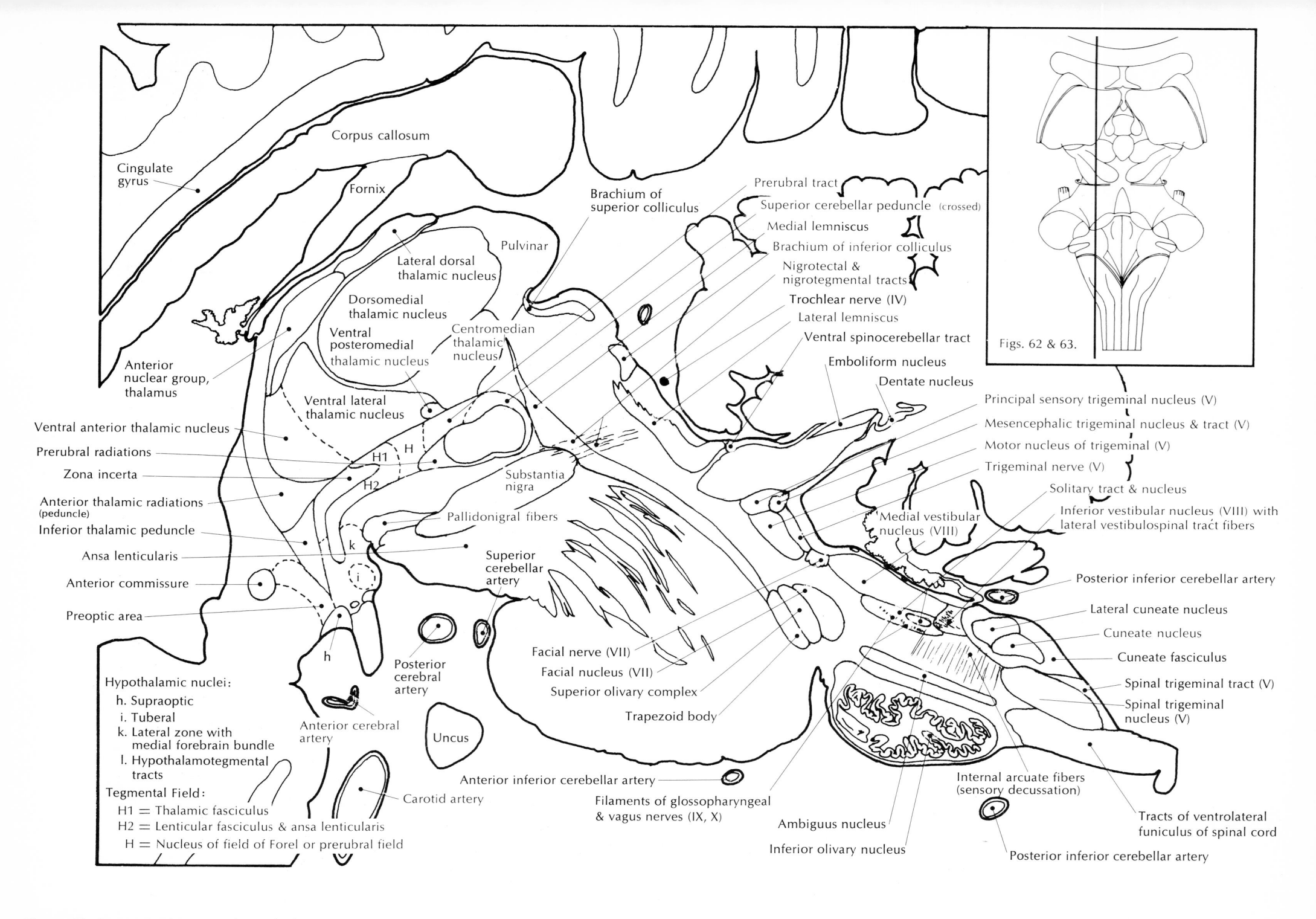

Cingulate gyrus

Corpus callosum

Fornix

Brachium of superior colliculus

Prerubral tract

Superior cerebellar peduncle (crossed)

Medial lemniscus

Brachium of inferior colliculus

Nigrotectal & nigrotegmental tracts

Trochlear nerve (IV)

Lateral lemniscus

Ventral spinocerebellar tract

Figs. 62 & 63.

Lateral dorsal thalamic nucleus

Pulvinar

Dorsomedial thalamic nucleus

Ventral posteromedial thalamic nucleus

Centromedian thalamic nucleus

Emboliform nucleus

Dentate nucleus

Anterior nuclear group, thalamus

Ventral lateral thalamic nucleus

Principal sensory trigeminal nucleus (V)

Mesencephalic trigeminal nucleus & tract (V)

Motor nucleus of trigeminal (V)

Trigeminal nerve (V)

Solitary tract & nucleus

Inferior vestibular nucleus (VIII) with lateral vestibulospinal tract fibers

Ventral anterior thalamic nucleus

Prerubral radiations

Zona incerta

H1 H

Substantia nigra

H2

Anterior thalamic radiations (peduncle)

Inferior thalamic peduncle

Pallidonigral fibers

Medial vestibular nucleus (VIII)

Ansa lenticularis

k

Posterior inferior cerebellar artery

Anterior commissure

i

Superior cerebellar artery

Lateral cuneate nucleus

Preoptic area

Cuneate nucleus

h

Cuneate fasciculus

Hypothalamic nuclei:

h. Supraoptic

i. Tuberal

k. Lateral zone with medial forebrain bundle

l. Hypothalamotegmental tracts

Posterior cerebral artery

Facial nerve (VII)

Facial nucleus (VII)

Superior olivary complex

Trapezoid body

Spinal trigeminal tract (V)

Spinal trigeminal nucleus (V)

Anterior cerebral artery

Uncus

Tegmental Field:

H1 = Thalamic fasciculus

H2 = Lenticular fasciculus & ansa lenticularis

H = Nucleus of field of Forel or prerubral field

Carotid artery

Anterior inferior cerebellar artery

Filaments of glossopharyngeal & vagus nerves (IX, X)

Ambiguus nucleus

Inferior olivary nucleus

Internal arcuate fibers (sensory decussation)

Tracts of ventrolateral funiculus of spinal cord

Posterior inferior cerebellar artery

Figure 62. Parasagittal section through the special visceral efferent cell column of the medulla and pons—Weil, 3.5X

124

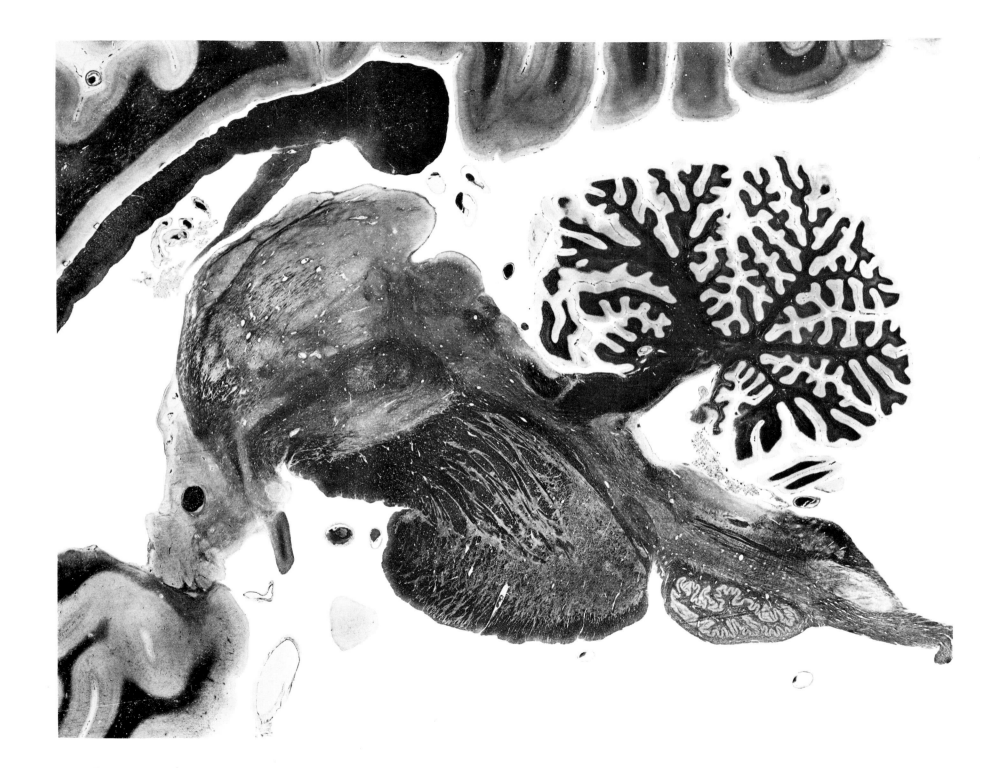

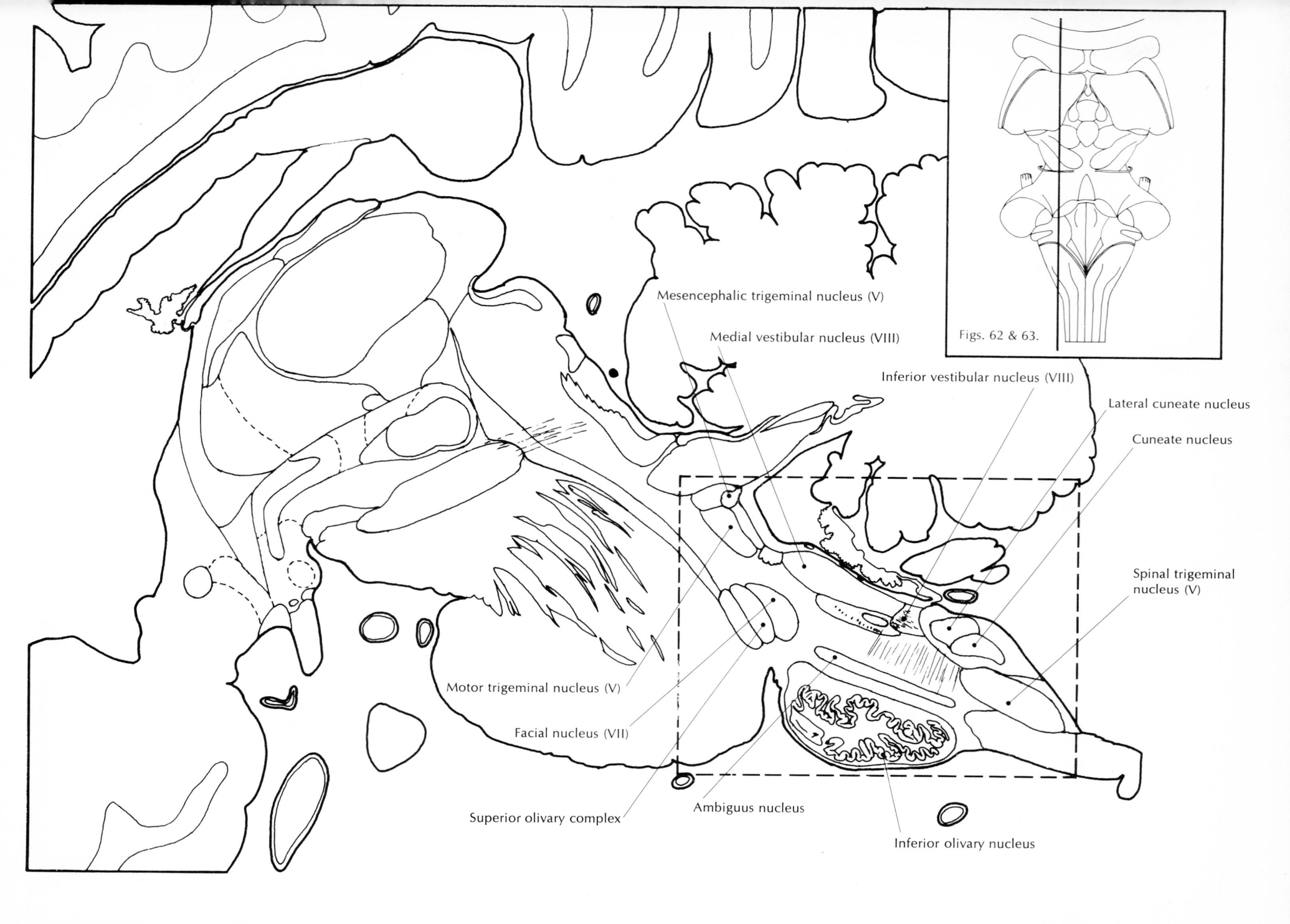

Mesencephalic trigeminal nucleus (V)

Medial vestibular nucleus (VIII)

Figs. 62 & 63.

Inferior vestibular nucleus (VIII)

Lateral cuneate nucleus

Cuneate nucleus

Spinal trigeminal nucleus (V)

Motor trigeminal nucleus (V)

Facial nucleus (VII)

Superior olivary complex

Ambiguus nucleus

Inferior olivary nucleus

Figure 63. Detail of the special visceral efferent cell column in the pons and medulla— Nissl, 11X

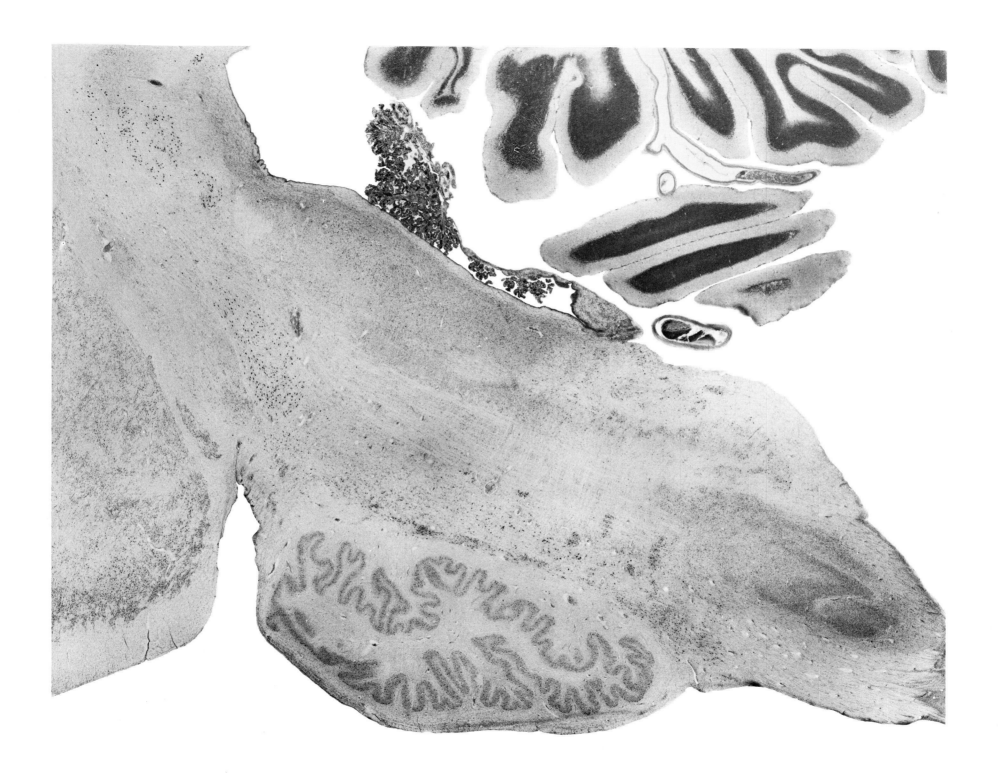

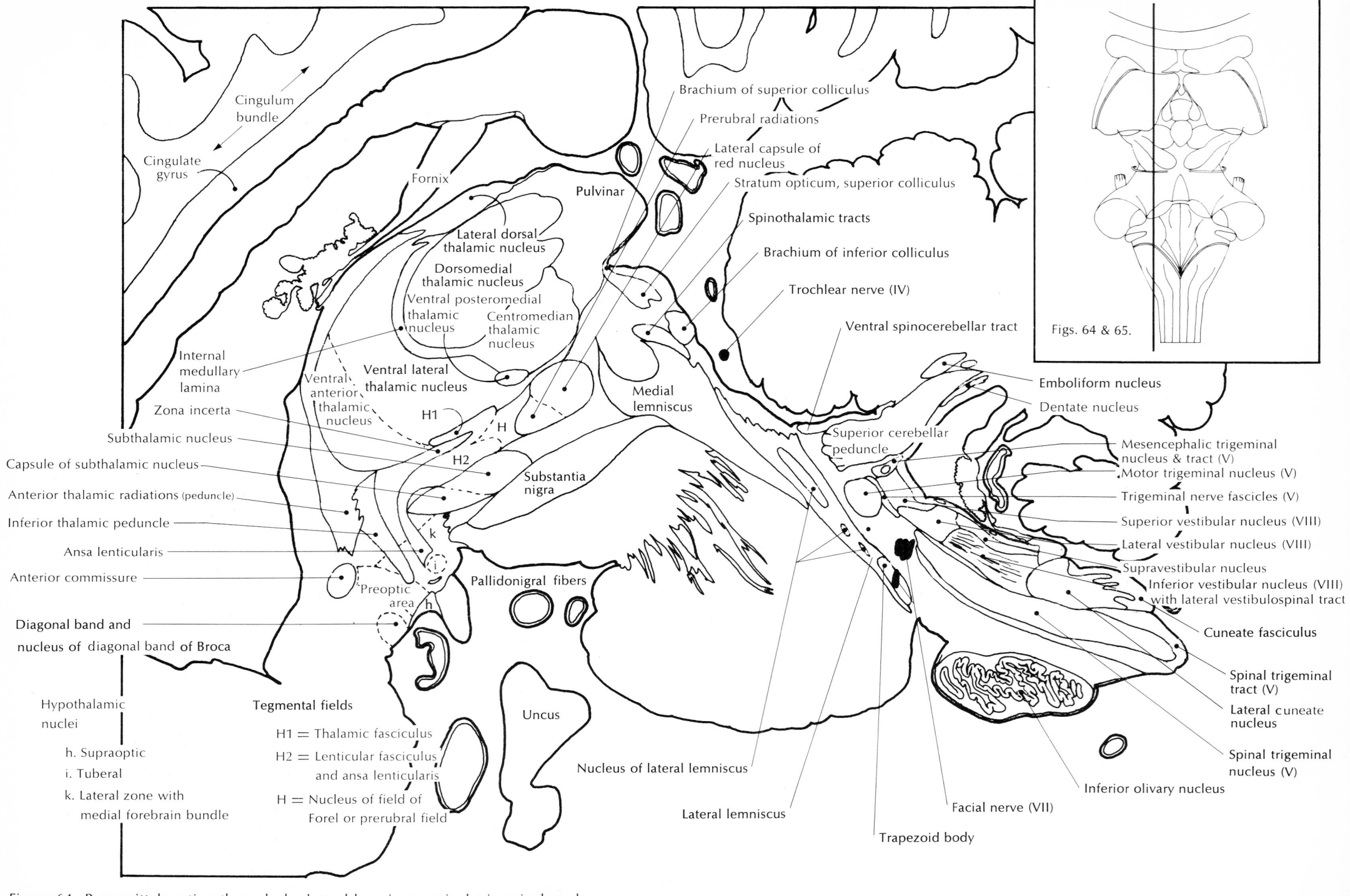

Figure 64. Parasagittal section through the lateral lemniscus, spinal trigeminal nucleus, and lateral vestibulospinal tract—Weil, 3.5X

128

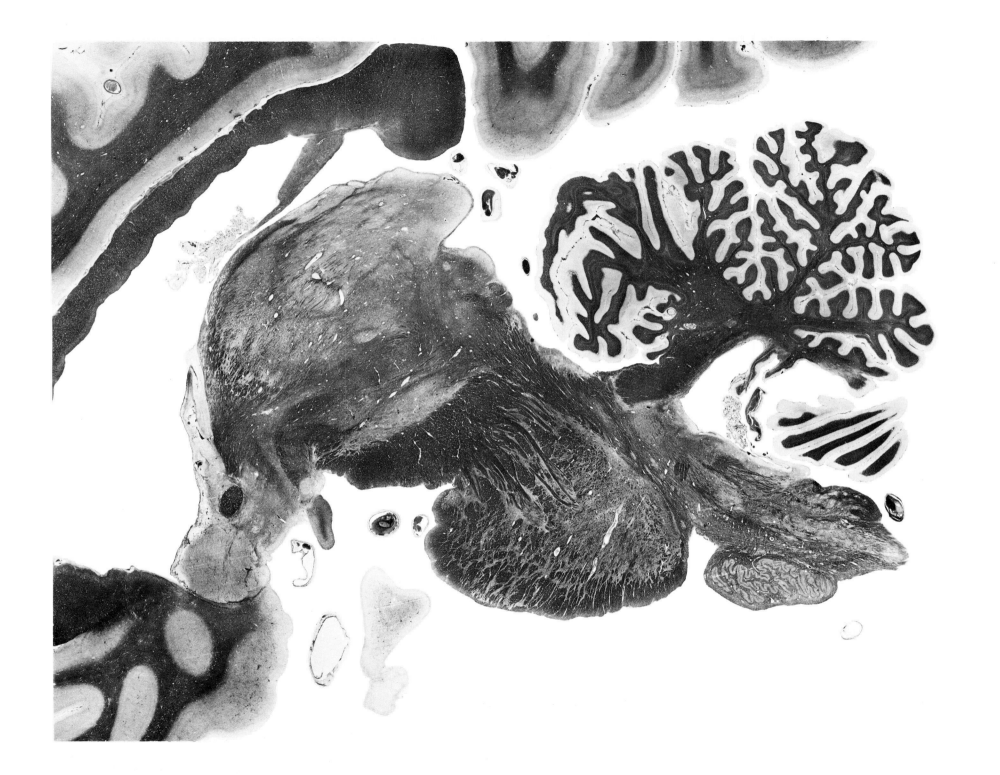

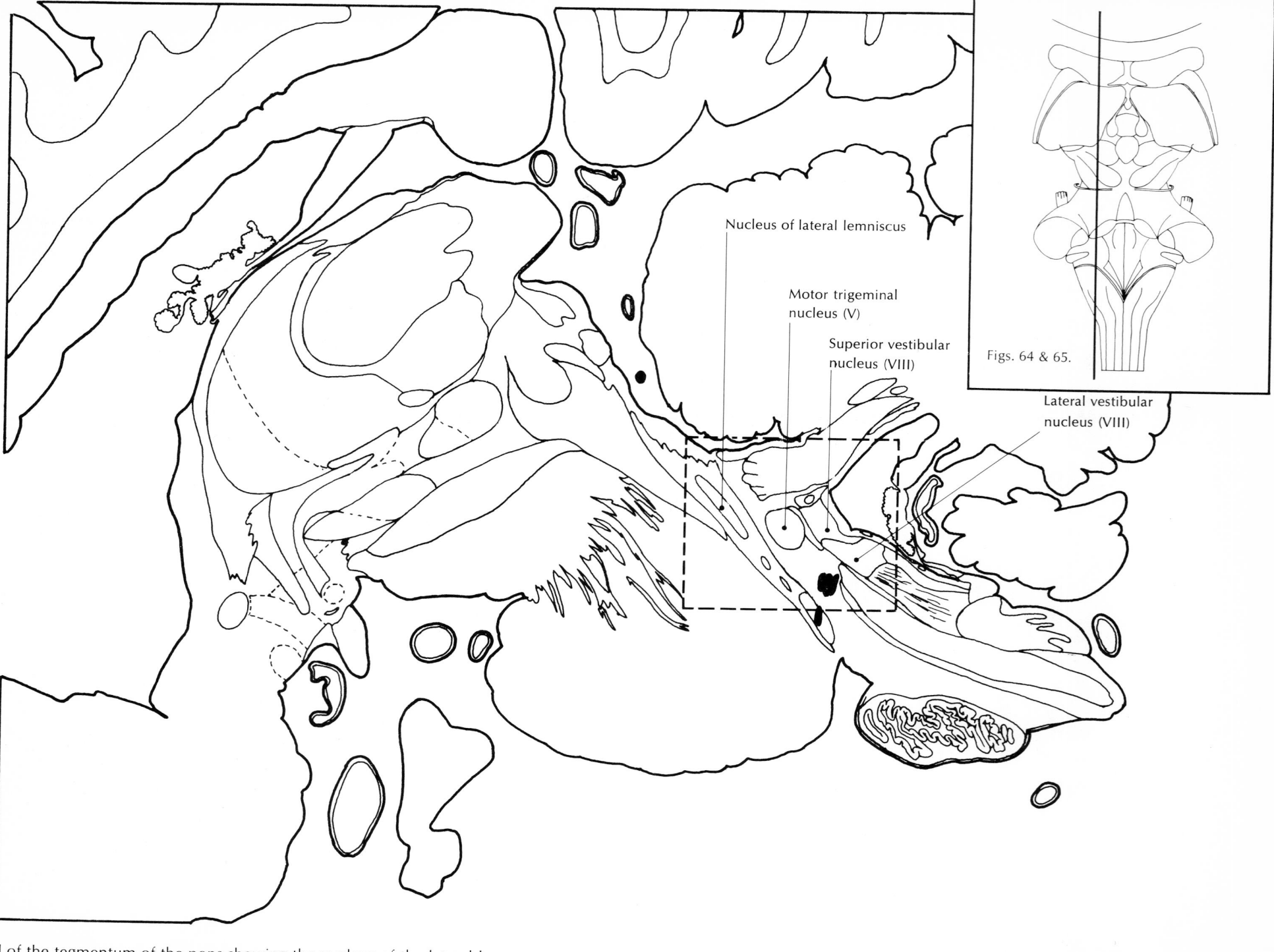

Nucleus of lateral lemniscus

Motor trigeminal
nucleus (V)

Superior vestibular
nucleus (VIII)

Figs. 64 & 65.

Lateral vestibular
nucleus (VIII)

Figure 65. Detail of the tegmentum of the pons showing the nucleus of the lateral lemniscus coursing obliquely within the lateral lemniscus—Nissl, 30X

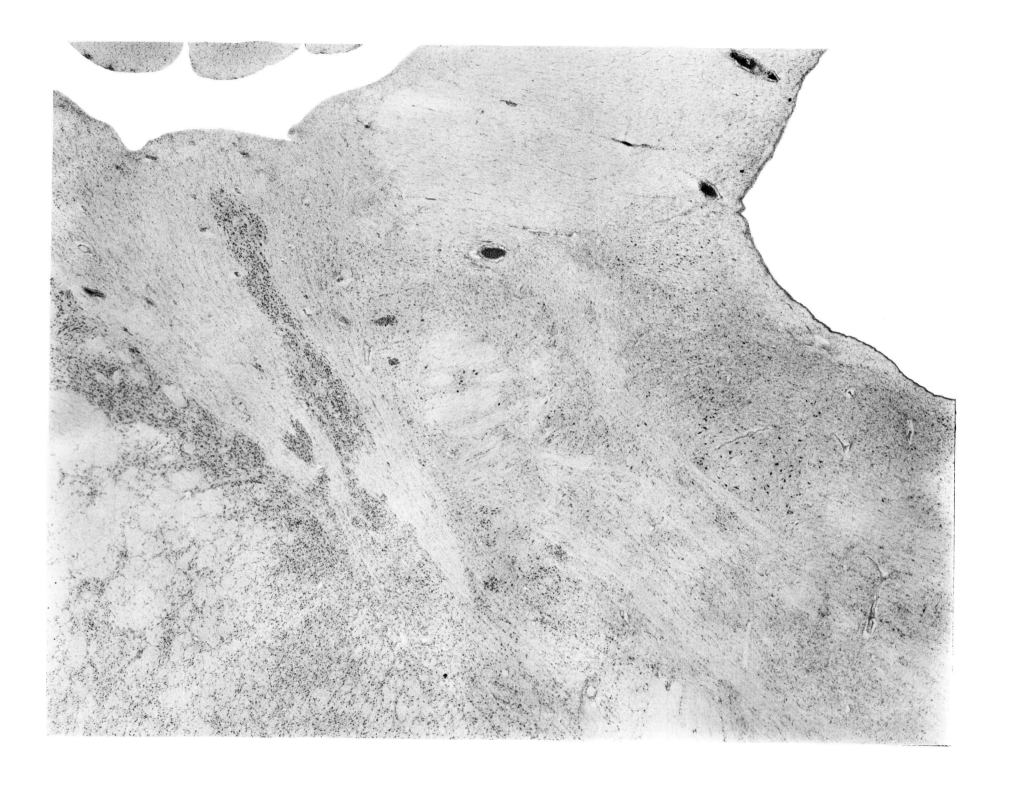

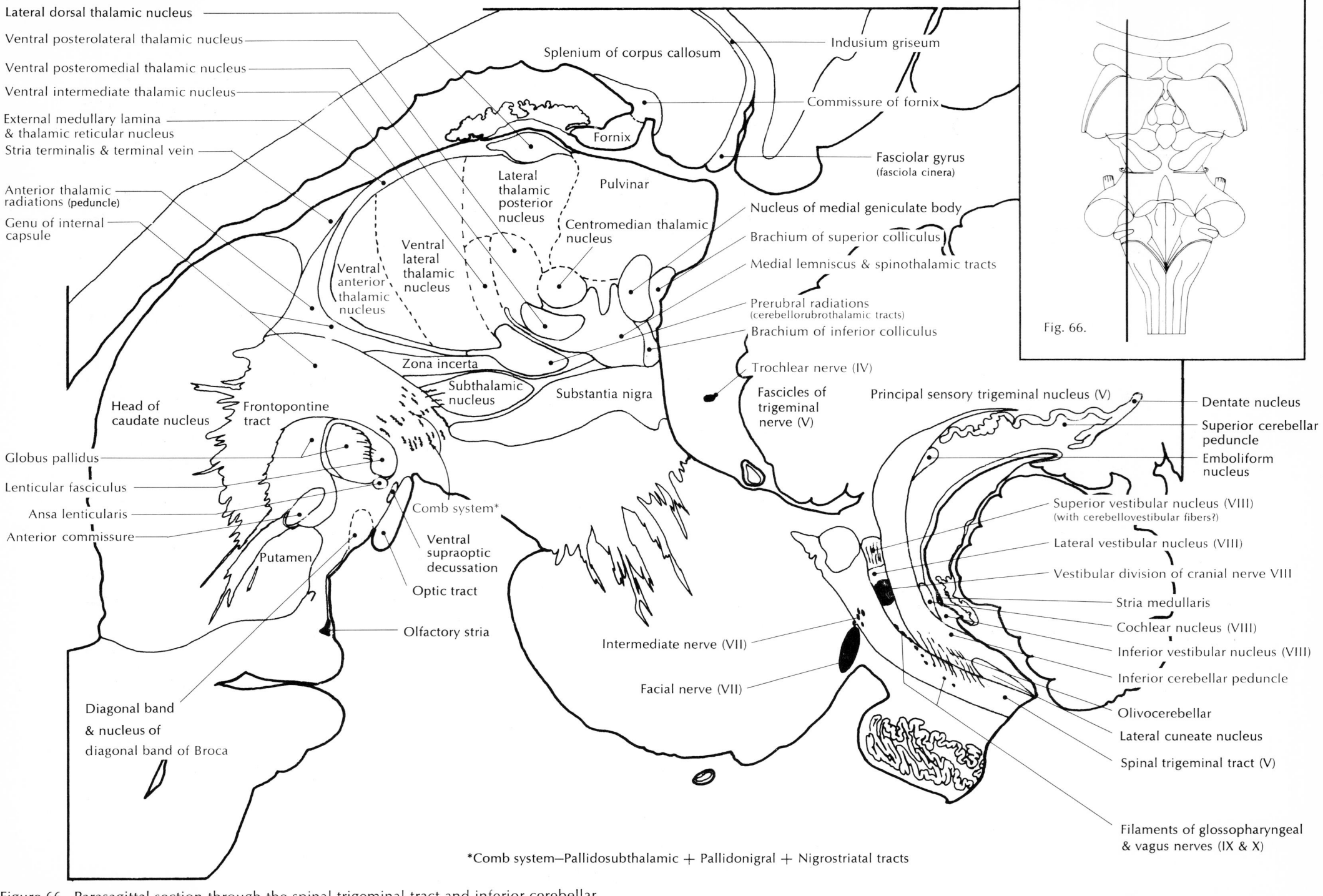

Lateral dorsal thalamic nucleus

Ventral posterolateral thalamic nucleus

Ventral posteromedial thalamic nucleus

Ventral intermediate thalamic nucleus

External medullary lamina & thalamic reticular nucleus

Stria terminalis & terminal vein

Anterior thalamic radiations (peduncle)

Genu of internal capsule

Anterior thalamic nucleus

Head of caudate nucleus

Frontopontine tract

Globus pallidus

Lenticular fasciculus

Ansa lenticularis

Anterior commissure

Putamen

Diagonal band & nucleus of diagonal band of Broca

Ventral anterior thalamic nucleus

Ventral lateral thalamic nucleus

Lateral thalamic posterior nucleus

Centromedian thalamic nucleus

Zona incerta

Subthalamic nucleus

Comb system*

Ventral supraoptic decussation

Optic tract

Olfactory stria

Splenium of corpus callosum

Fornix

Pulvinar

Substantia nigra

Indusium griseum

Commissure of fornix

Fasciolar gyrus (fasciola cinera)

Nucleus of medial geniculate body

Brachium of superior colliculus

Medial lemniscus & spinothalamic tracts

Prerubral radiations (cerebellorubrothalamic tracts)

Brachium of inferior colliculus

Trochlear nerve (IV)

Fascicles of trigeminal nerve (V)

Principal sensory trigeminal nucleus (V)

Intermediate nerve (VII)

Facial nerve (VII)

Dentate nucleus

Superior cerebellar peduncle

Emboliform nucleus

Superior vestibular nucleus (VIII) (with cerebellovestibular fibers?)

Lateral vestibular nucleus (VIII)

Vestibular division of cranial nerve VIII

Stria medullaris

Cochlear nucleus (VIII)

Inferior vestibular nucleus (VIII)

Inferior cerebellar peduncle

Olivocerebellar

Lateral cuneate nucleus

Spinal trigeminal tract (V)

Filaments of glossopharyngeal & vagus nerves (IX & X)

Fig. 66.

*Comb system—Pallidosubthalamic + Pallidonigral + Nigrostriatal tracts

Figure 66. Parasagittal section through the spinal trigeminal tract and inferior cerebellar peduncle—Weil, 3.5X

132

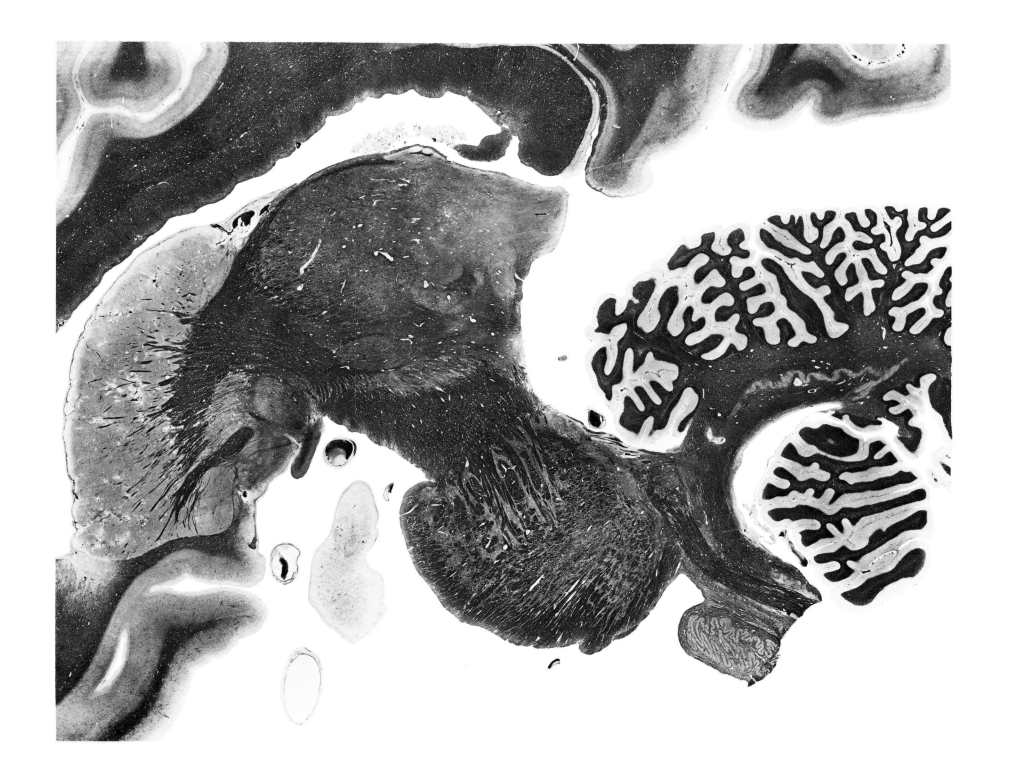

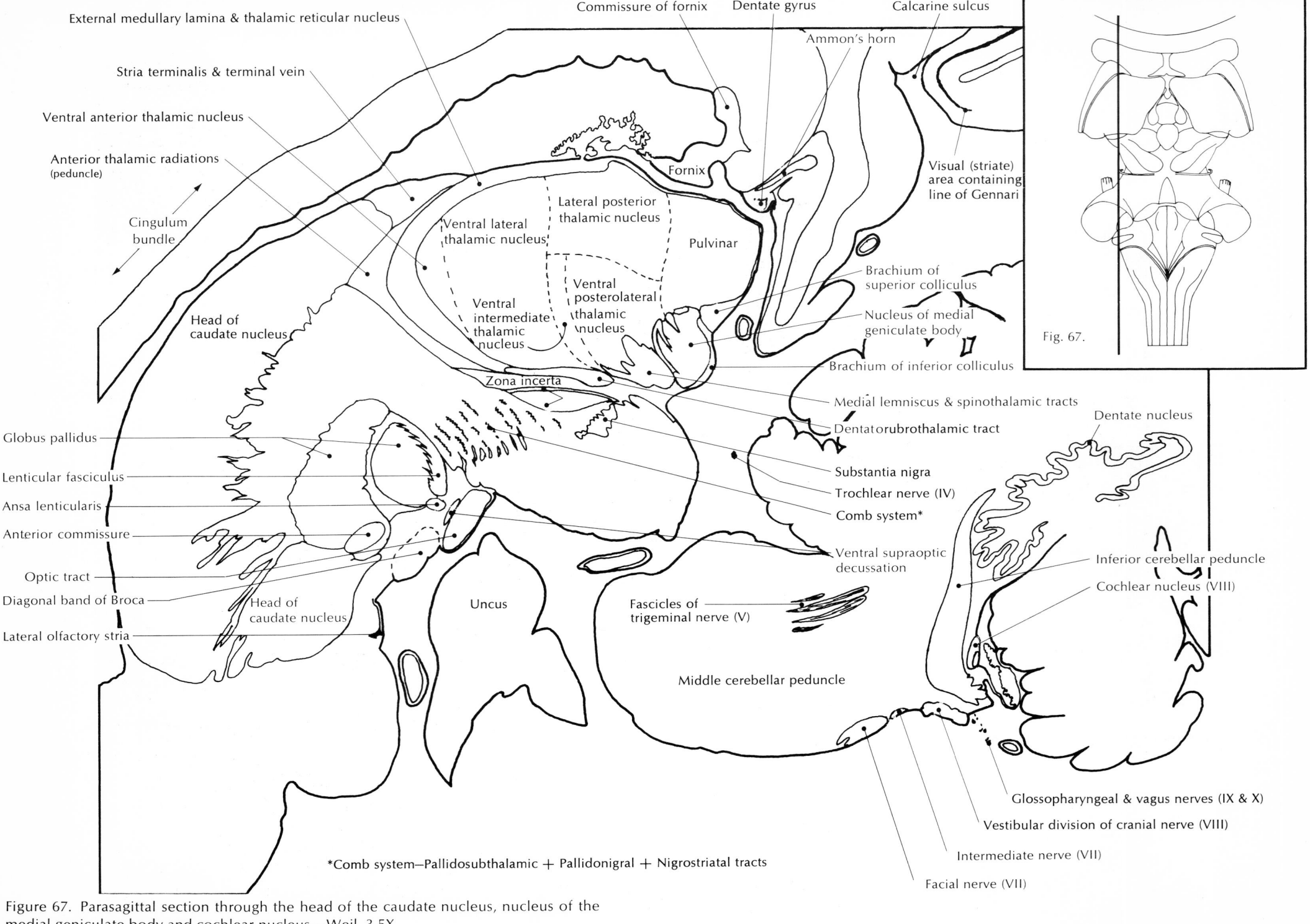

External medullary lamina & thalamic reticular nucleus

Stria terminalis & terminal vein

Ventral anterior thalamic nucleus

Anterior thalamic radiations
(peduncle)

Cingulum
bundle

Head of
caudate nucleus

Globus pallidus

Lenticular fasciculus

Ansa lenticularis

Anterior commissure

Optic tract

Diagonal band of Broca

Lateral olfactory stria

Head of
caudate nucleus

Uncus

Commissure of fornix

Dentate gyrus

Calcarine sulcus

Ammon's horn

Fornix

Lateral posterior
thalamic nucleus

Ventral lateral
thalamic nucleus

Pulvinar

Ventral
posterolateral
thalamic
nucleus

Ventral
intermediate
thalamic
nucleus

Zona incerta

Visual (striate)
area containing
line of Gennari

Fig. 67.

Brachium of
superior colliculus

Nucleus of medial
geniculate body

Brachium of inferior colliculus

Medial lemniscus & spinothalamic tracts

Dentatorubrothalamic tract

Substantia nigra

Trochlear nerve (IV)

Comb system*

Ventral supraoptic
decussation

Fascicles of
trigeminal nerve (V)

Dentate nucleus

Inferior cerebellar peduncle

Cochlear nucleus (VIII)

Middle cerebellar peduncle

Glossopharyngeal & vagus nerves (IX & X)

Vestibular division of cranial nerve (VIII)

Intermediate nerve (VII)

Facial nerve (VII)

*Comb system—Pallidosubthalamic + Pallidonigral + Nigrostriatal tracts

Figure 67. Parasagittal section through the head of the caudate nucleus, nucleus of the
medial geniculate body and cochlear nucleus—Weil, 3.5X

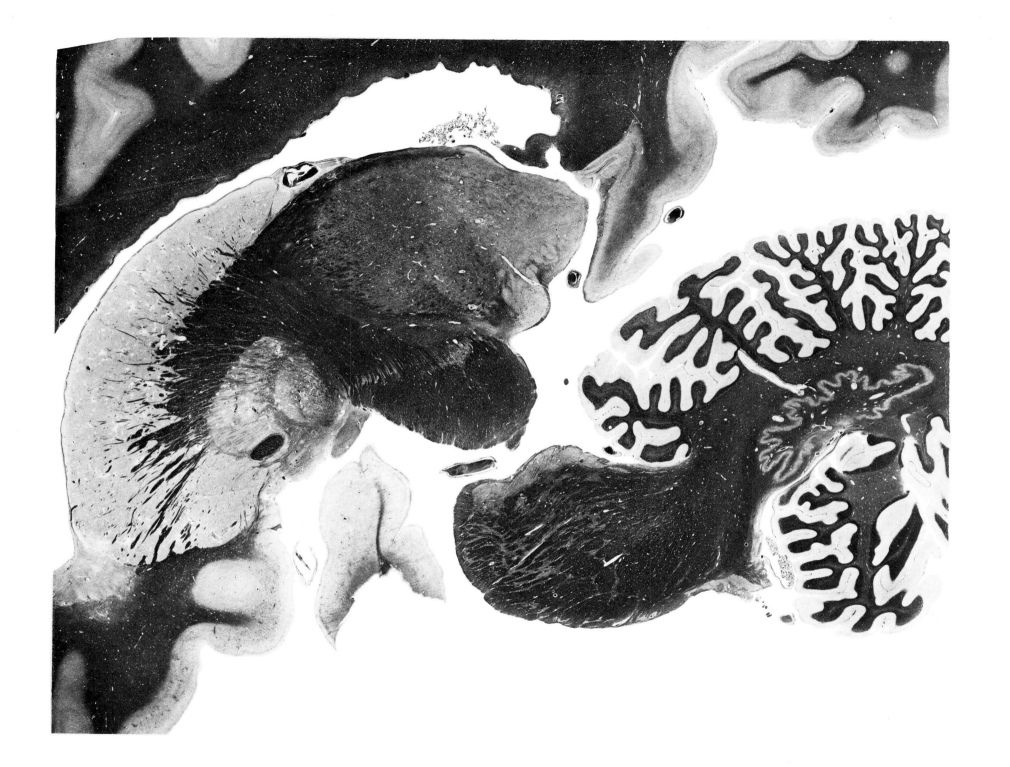

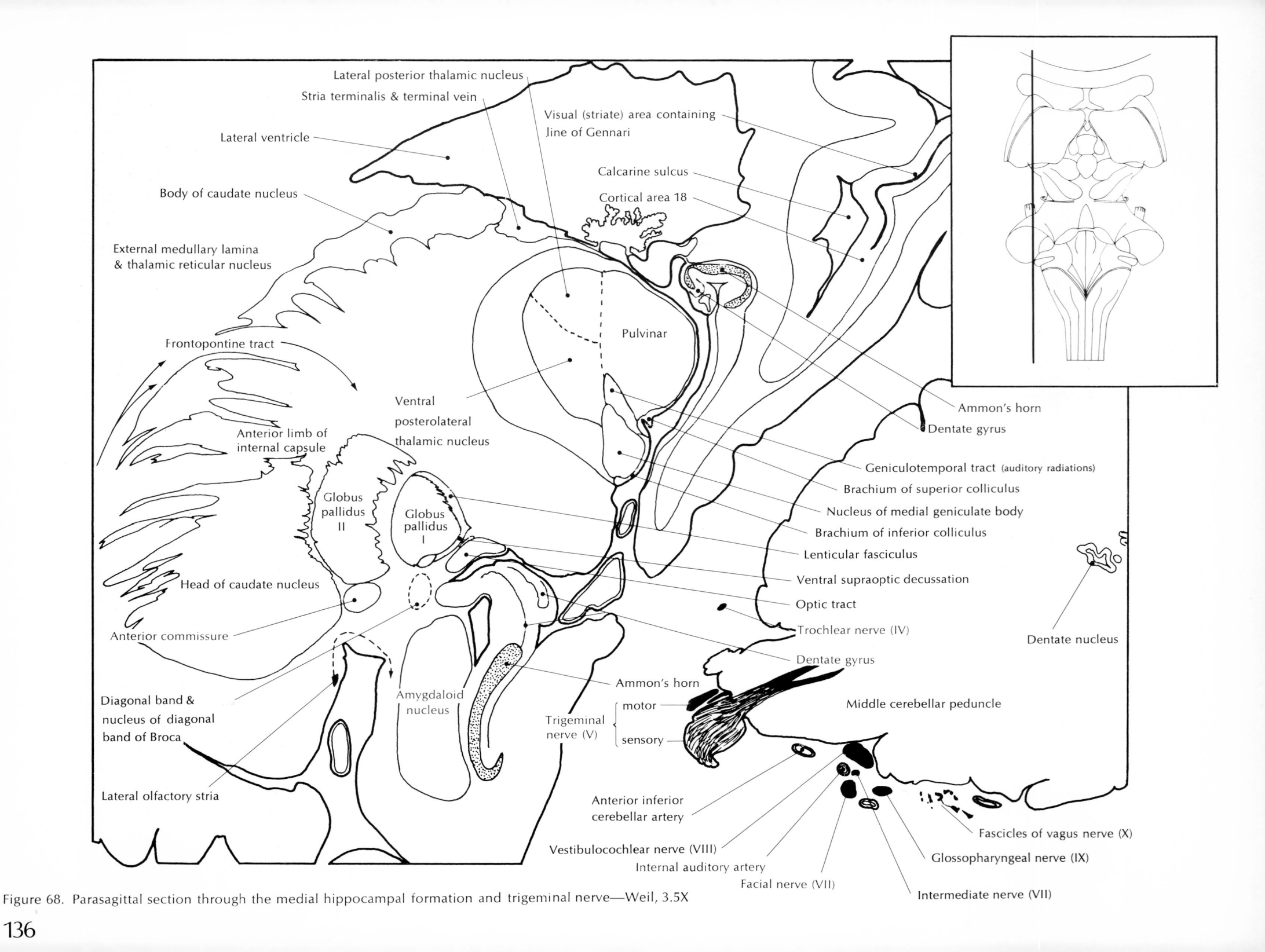

Figure 68. Parasagittal section through the medial hippocampal formation and trigeminal nerve—Weil, 3.5X

136

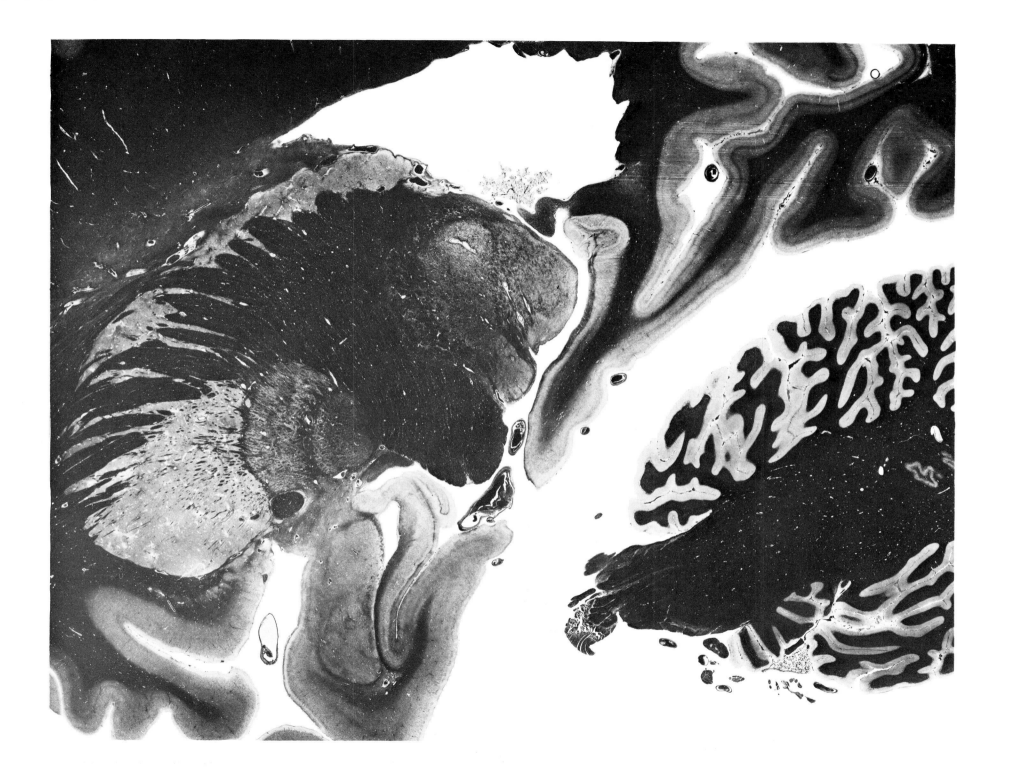

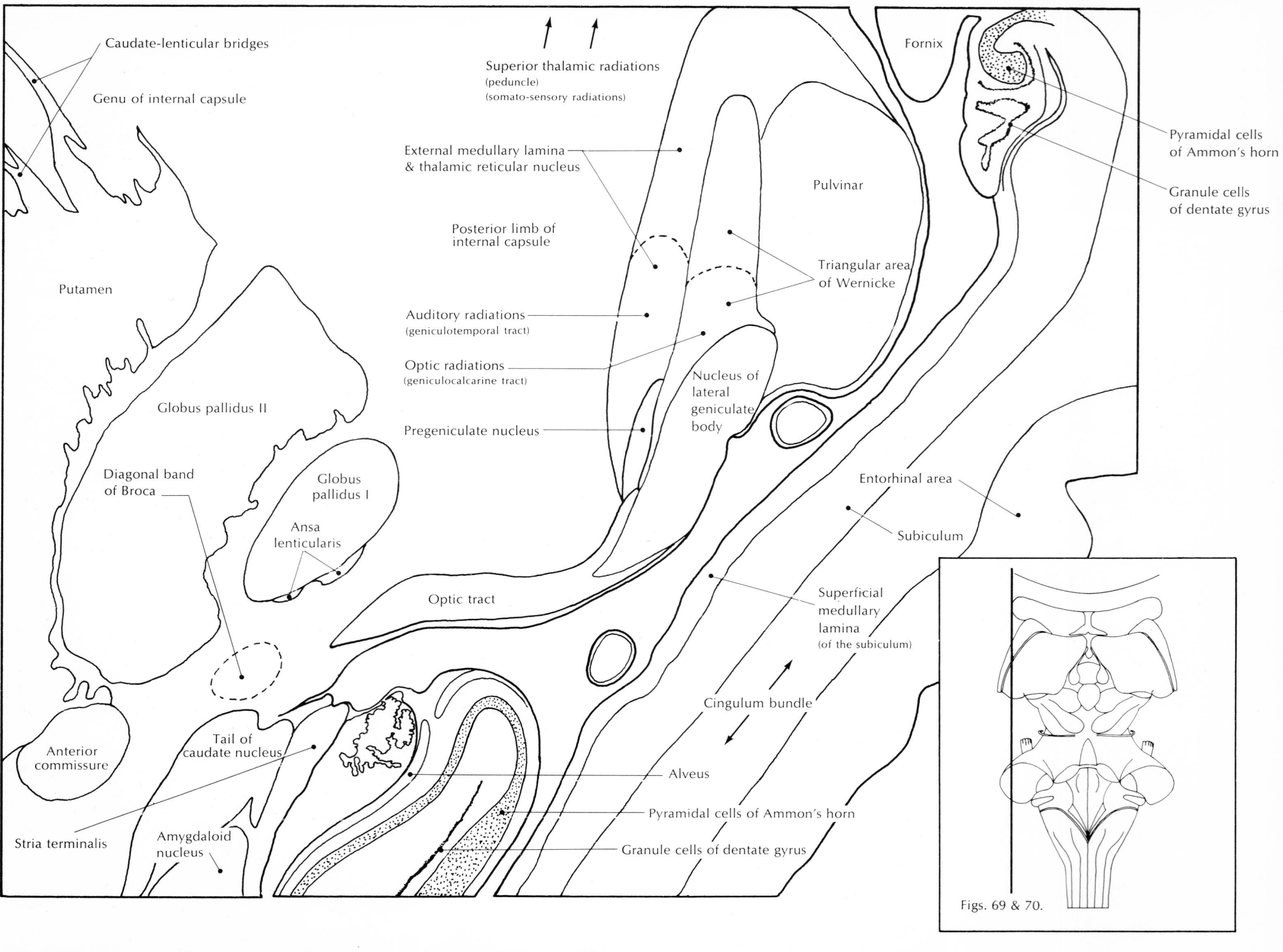

Figure 69. Parasagittal section through the nucleus of the lateral geniculate body—-Weil, 10X

Caudate-lenticular bridges

Genu of internal capsule

Putamen

Globus pallidus II

Diagonal band of Broca

Globus pallidus I

Ansa lenticularis

Optic tract

Anterior commissure

Tail of caudate nucleus

Stria terminalis

Amygdaloid nucleus

Superior thalamic radiations (peduncle) (somato-sensory radiations)

External medullary lamina & thalamic reticular nucleus

Posterior limb of internal capsule

Auditory radiations (geniculotemporal tract)

Optic radiations (geniculocalcarine tract)

Pregeniculate nucleus

Triangular area of Wernicke

Nucleus of lateral geniculate body

Pulvinar

Fornix

Pyramidal cells of Ammon's horn

Granule cells of dentate gyrus

Entorhinal area

Subiculum

Superficial medullary lamina (of the subiculum)

Cingulum bundle

Alveus

Pyramidal cells of Ammon's horn

Granule cells of dentate gyrus

Figs. 69 & 70.

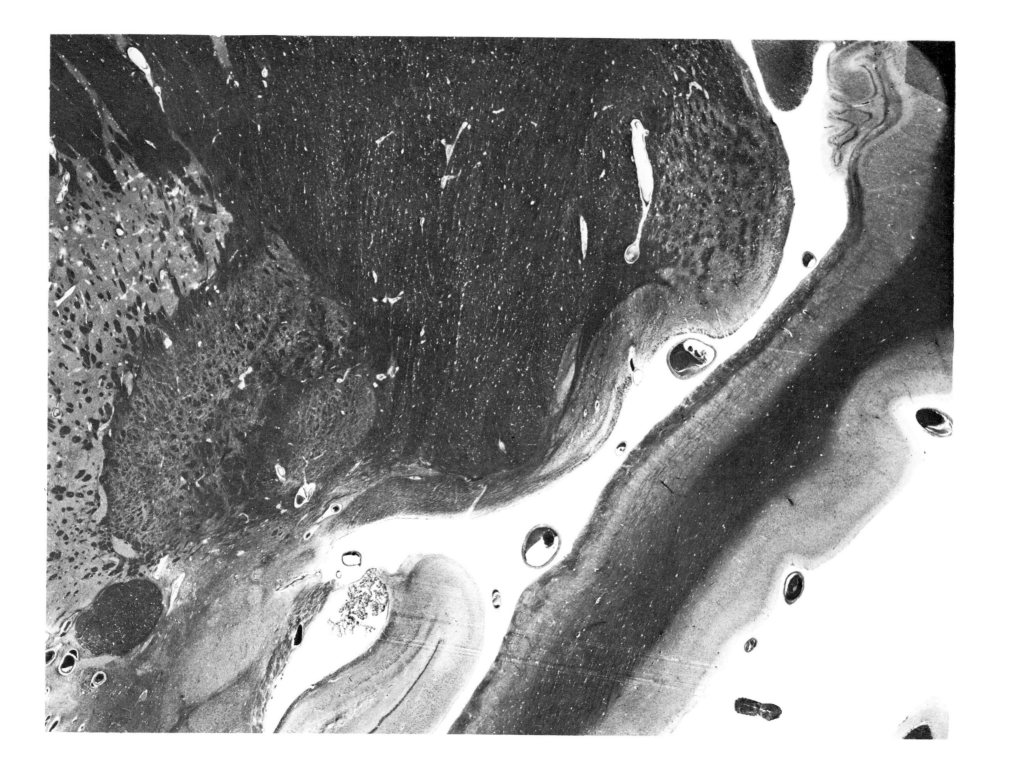

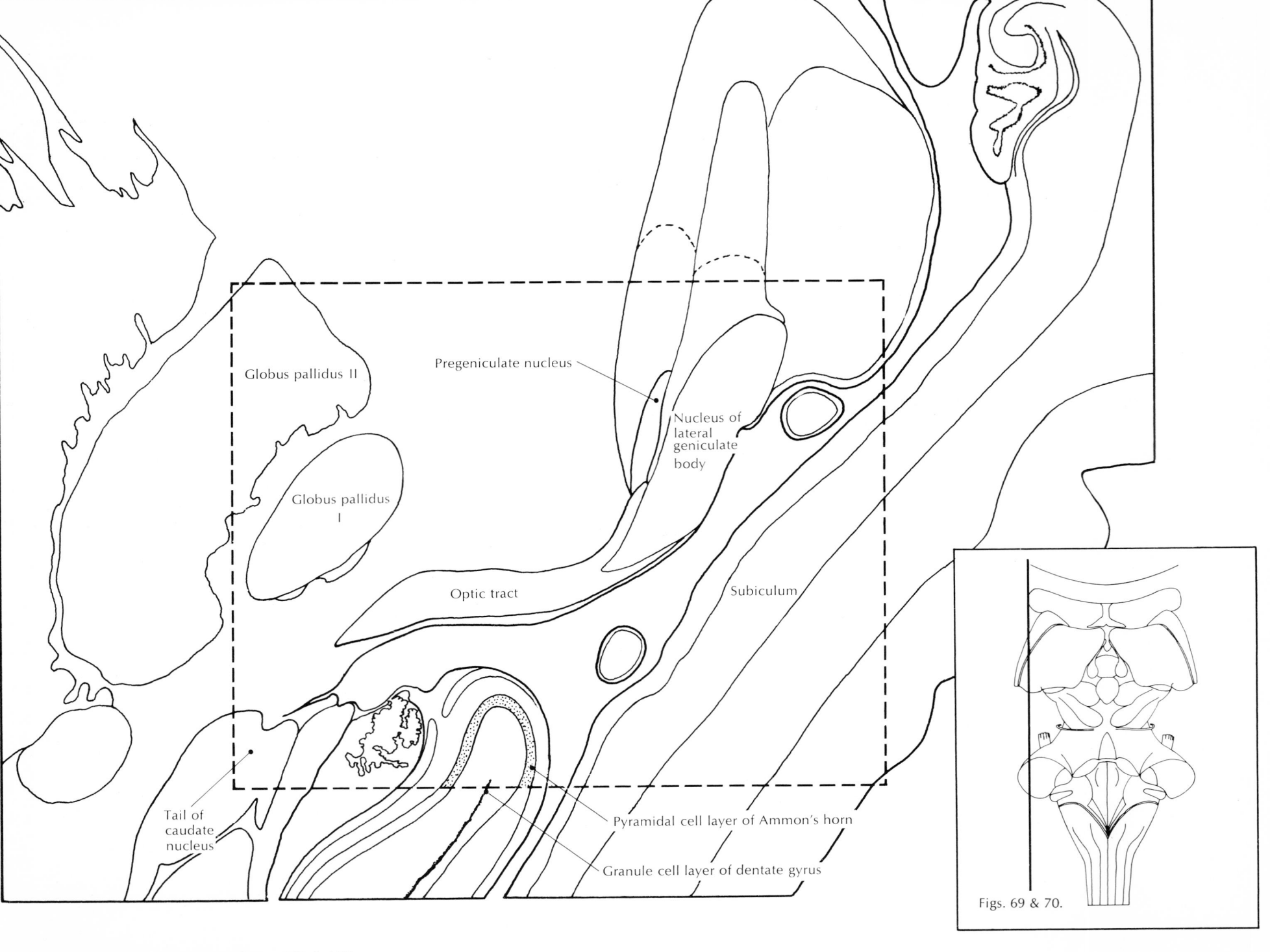

Figure 70. Detail of the lateral geniculate nucleus—Nissl, 17X

Globus pallidus II

Pregeniculate nucleus

Nucleus of lateral geniculate body

Globus pallidus I

Optic tract

Subiculum

Tail of caudate nucleus

Pyramidal cell layer of Ammon's horn

Granule cell layer of dentate gyrus

Figs. 69 & 70.

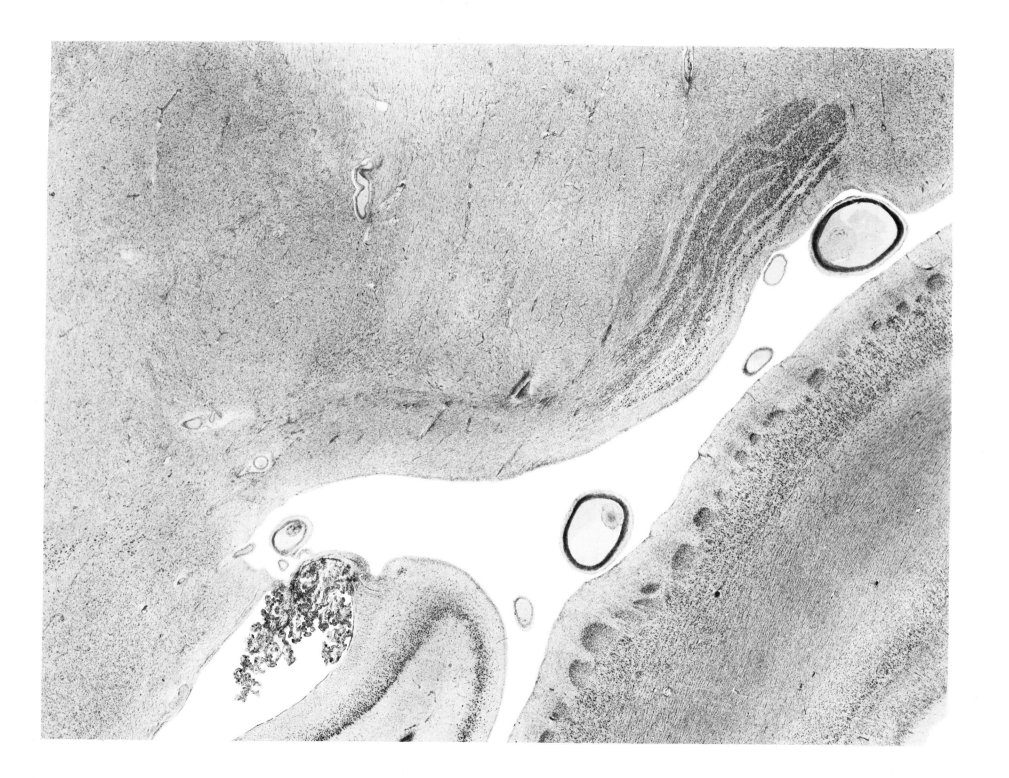

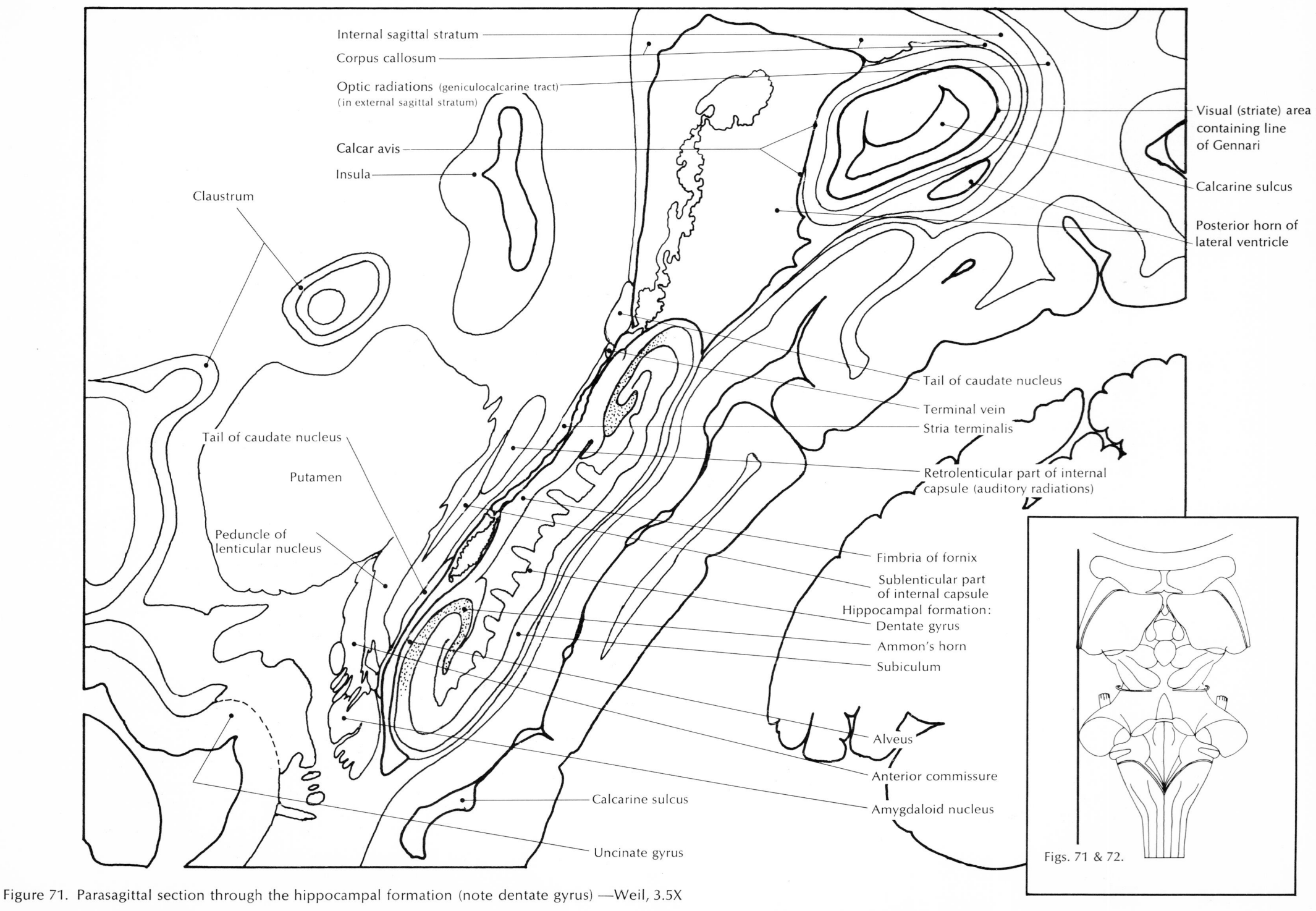

Internal sagittal stratum

Corpus callosum

Optic radiations (geniculocalcarine tract)
(in external sagittal stratum)

Calcar avis

Insula

Claustrum

Tail of caudate nucleus

Putamen

Peduncle of
lenticular nucleus

Visual (striate) area
containing line
of Gennari

Calcarine sulcus

Posterior horn of
lateral ventricle

Tail of caudate nucleus

Terminal vein

Stria terminalis

Retrolenticular part of internal
capsule (auditory radiations)

Fimbria of fornix

Sublenticular part
of internal capsule

Hippocampal formation:
Dentate gyrus

Ammon's horn

Subiculum

Alveus

Anterior commissure

Amygdaloid nucleus

Calcarine sulcus

Uncinate gyrus

Figs. 71 & 72.

Figure 71. Parasagittal section through the hippocampal formation (note dentate gyrus) —Weil, 3.5X

142

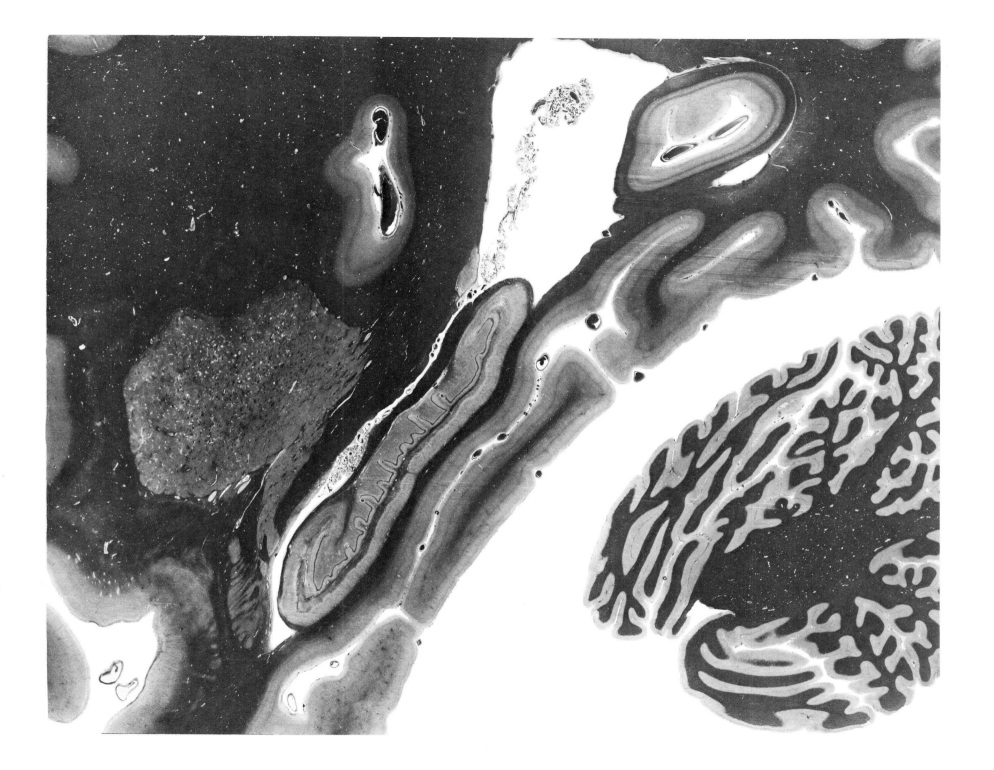

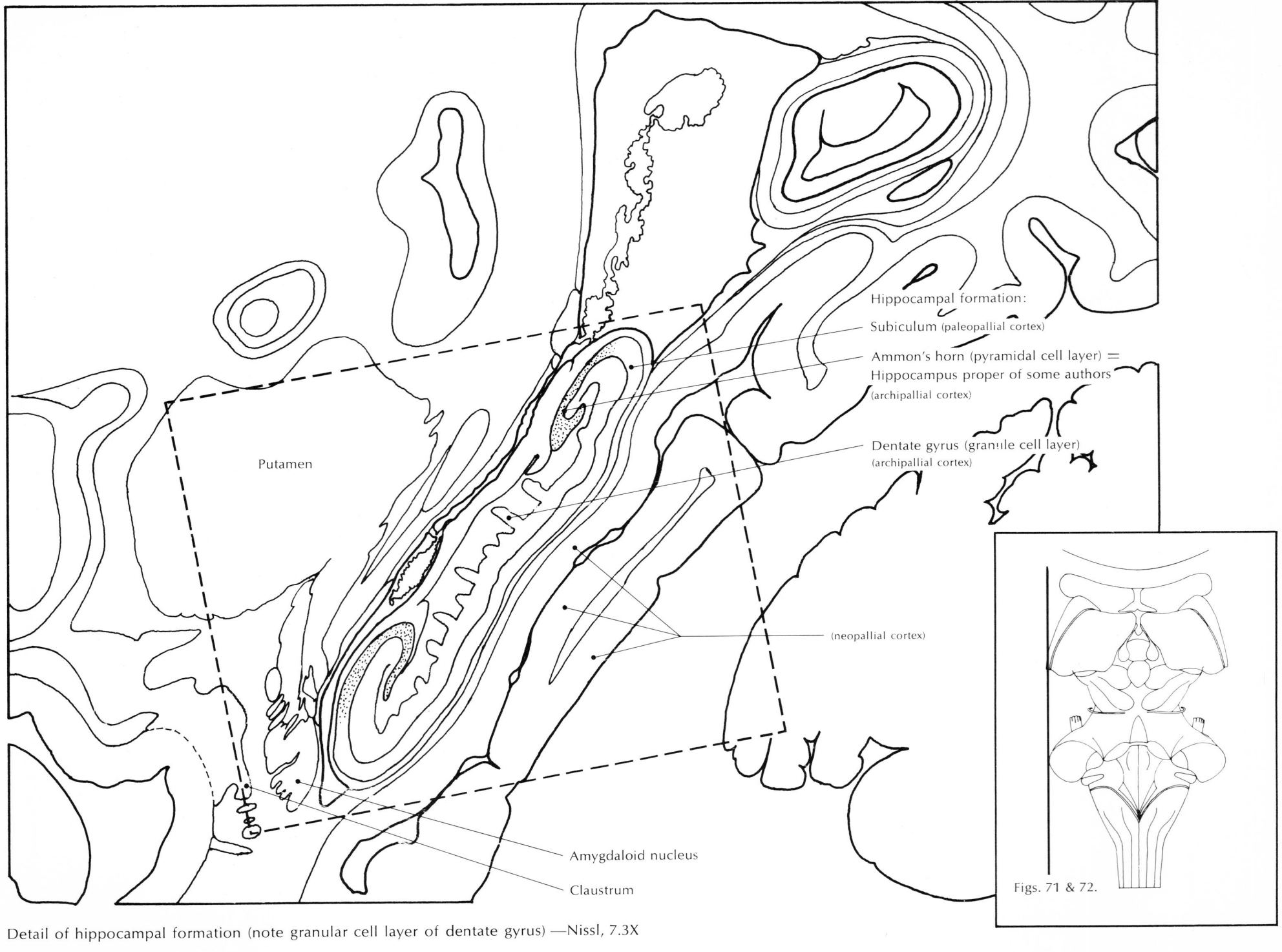

Hippocampal formation:

Subiculum (paleopallial cortex)

Ammon's horn (pyramidal cell layer) =
Hippocampus proper of some authors
(archipallial cortex)

Dentate gyrus (granule cell layer)
(archipallial cortex)

Putamen

(neopallial cortex)

Amygdaloid nucleus

Claustrum

Figs. 71 & 72.

Figure 72. Detail of hippocampal formation (note granular cell layer of dentate gyrus) —Nissl, 7.3X

144

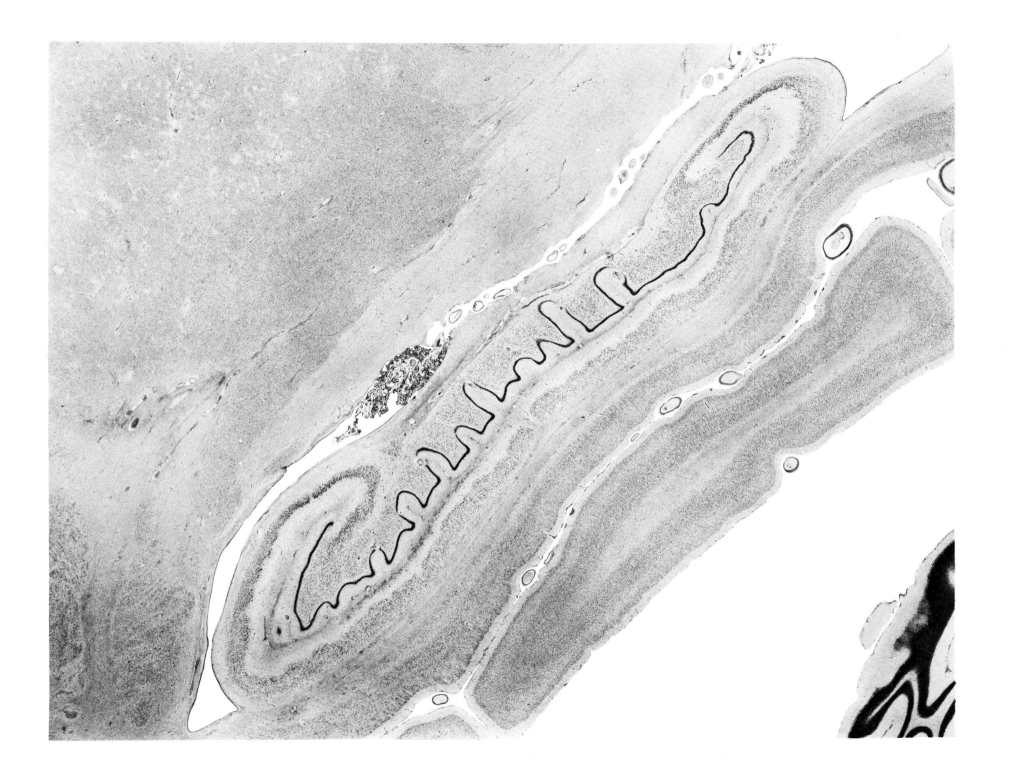

CYTOARCHITECTURE OF THE CEREBRAL CORTEX

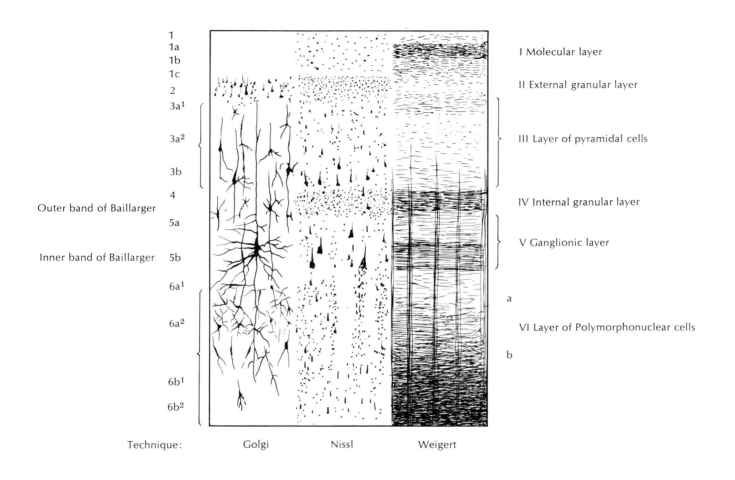

1
1a
1b
1c
2
3a¹
3a²
3b
4
Outer band of Baillarger
5a
Inner band of Baillarger   5b
6a¹
6a²
6b¹
6b²

I Molecular layer

II External granular layer

III Layer of pyramidal cells

IV Internal granular layer

V Ganglionic layer

a

VI Layer of Polymorphonuclear cells

b

Technique: Golgi   Nissl   Weigert

Figure 73. Diagram of cerebral cortex architecture. In area 17 (primary visual cortex) the outer line of Baillarger is termed the line of Gennari and is visible to the naked eye. (From Brodmann.)

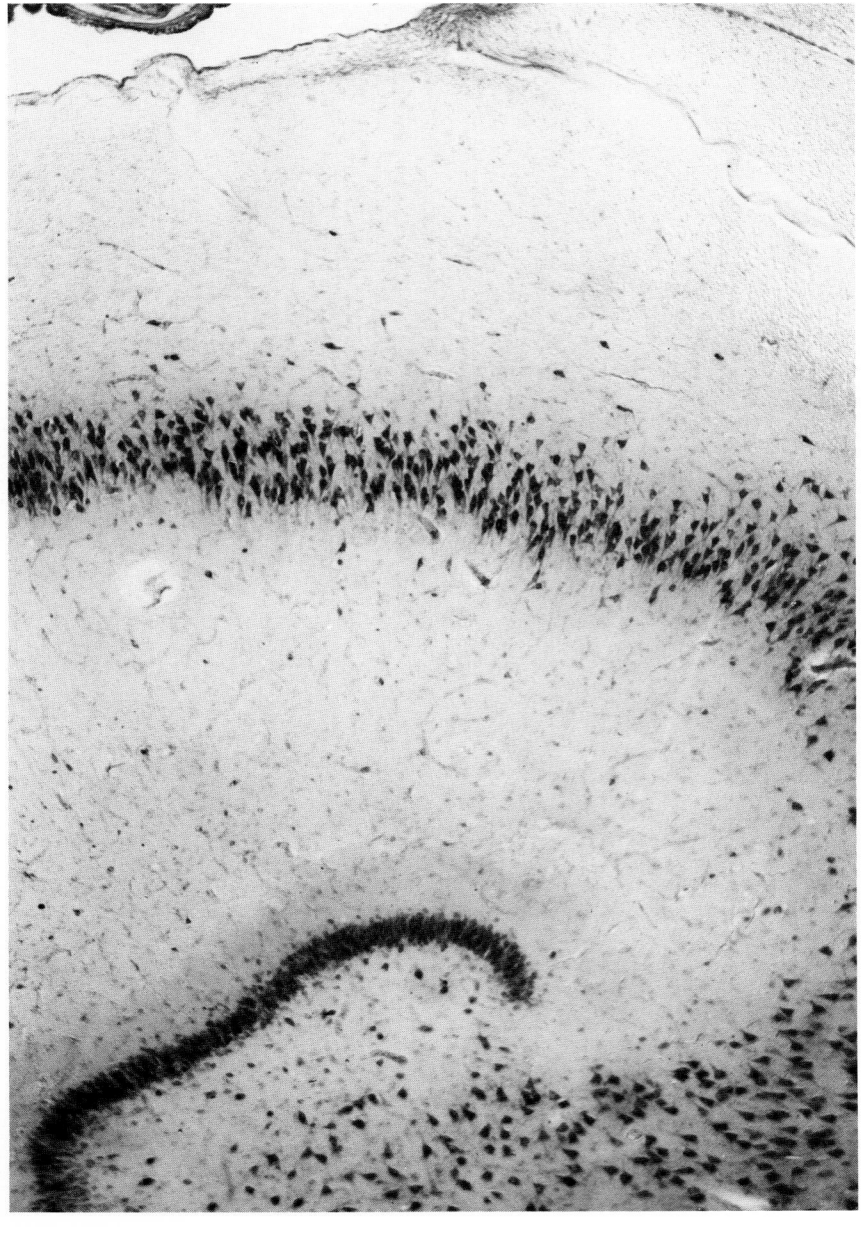

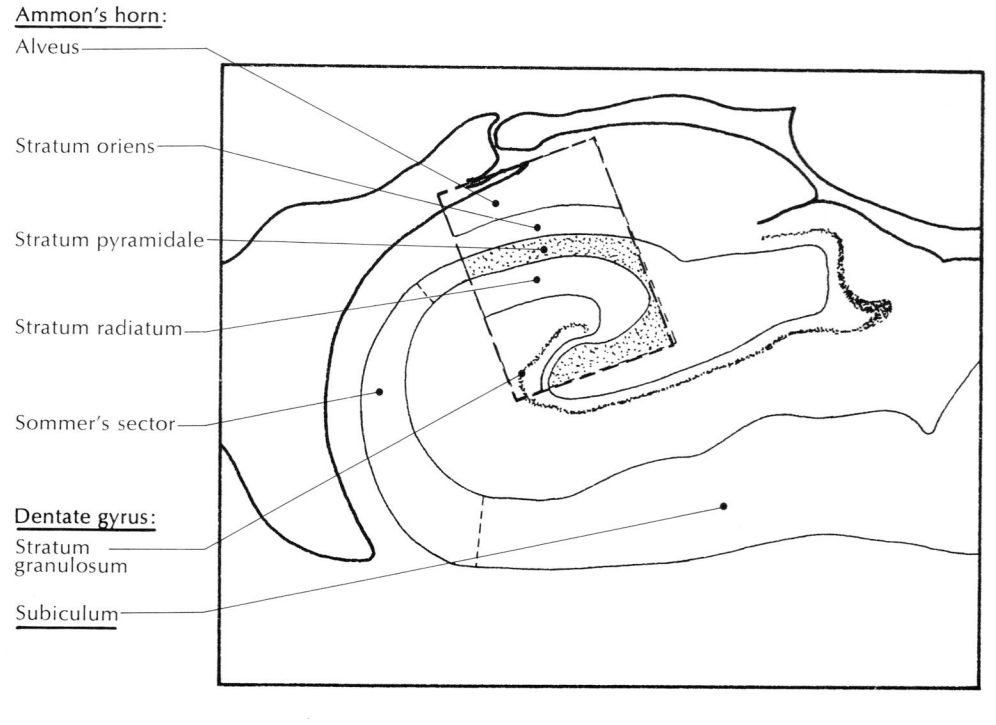

Figure 74. Allo- or heterogenetic cortex (e.g., hippocampal formation: dentate gyrus, Ammons horn, and subiculum). Photograph of pyramidal cell layer of Ammon's horn and granule cell layer of dentate gyrus—Nissl, 75X. Drawing of transverse section of hippocampal formation indicating layers or strata of Ammon's horn. Sommer's sector is the cellular area of Ammon's horn most sensitive to anoxia.

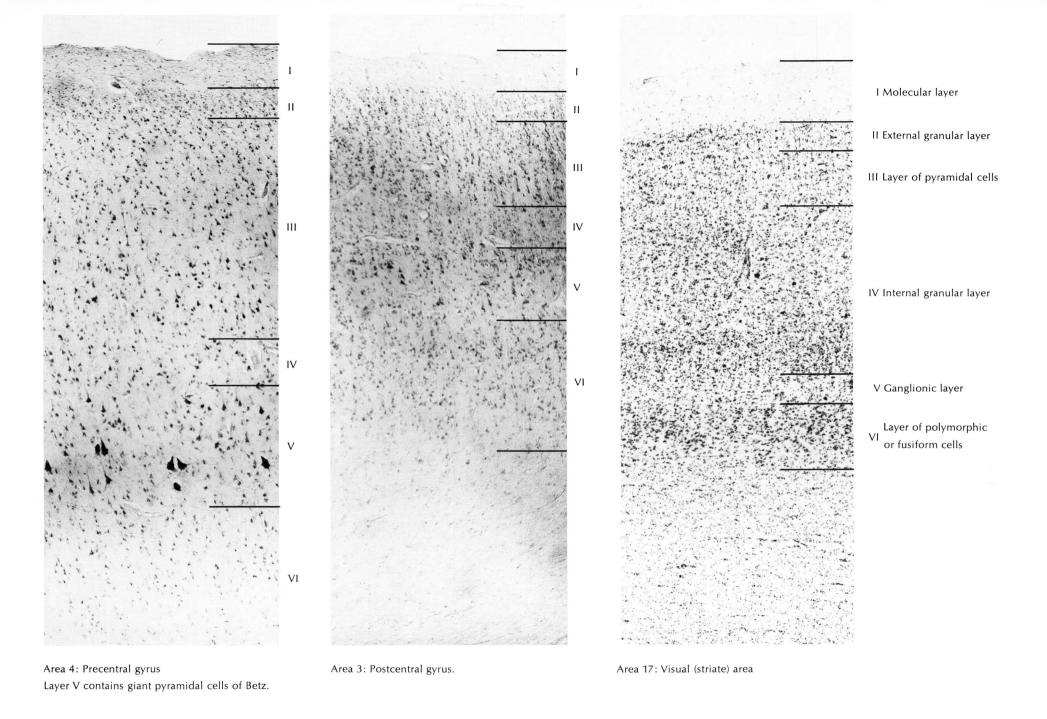

I

II

III

IV

V

VI

I

II

III

IV

V

VI

I Molecular layer

II External granular layer

III Layer of pyramidal cells

IV Internal granular layer

V Ganglionic layer

VI Layer of polymorphic or fusiform cells

Area 4: Precentral gyrus   Area 3: Postcentral gyrus.   Area 17: Visual (striate) area

Layer V contains giant pyramidal cells of Betz.

Figure 75. Iso- or homogenetic cortex (e.g., the six-layered cortex of the entire neopallium)—Nissl, 65X.

149

BLOOD SUPPLY OF THE BRAIN; ARTERIOGRAMS

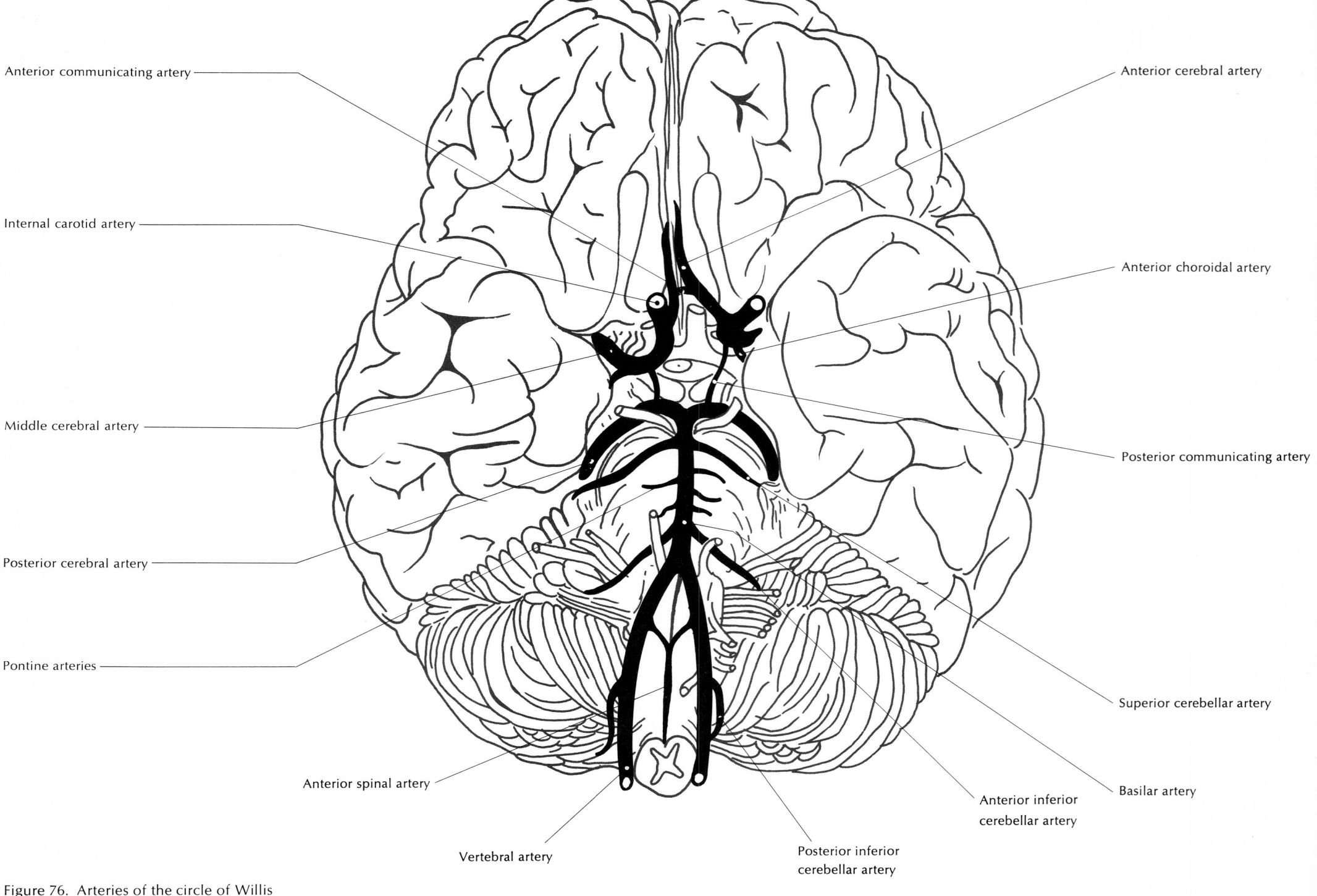

Anterior communicating artery

Internal carotid artery

Middle cerebral artery

Posterior cerebral artery

Pontine arteries

Anterior spinal artery

Vertebral artery

Posterior inferior
cerebellar artery

Anterior inferior
cerebellar artery

Basilar artery

Superior cerebellar artery

Posterior communicating artery

Anterior choroidal artery

Anterior cerebral artery

Figure 76. Arteries of the circle of Willis

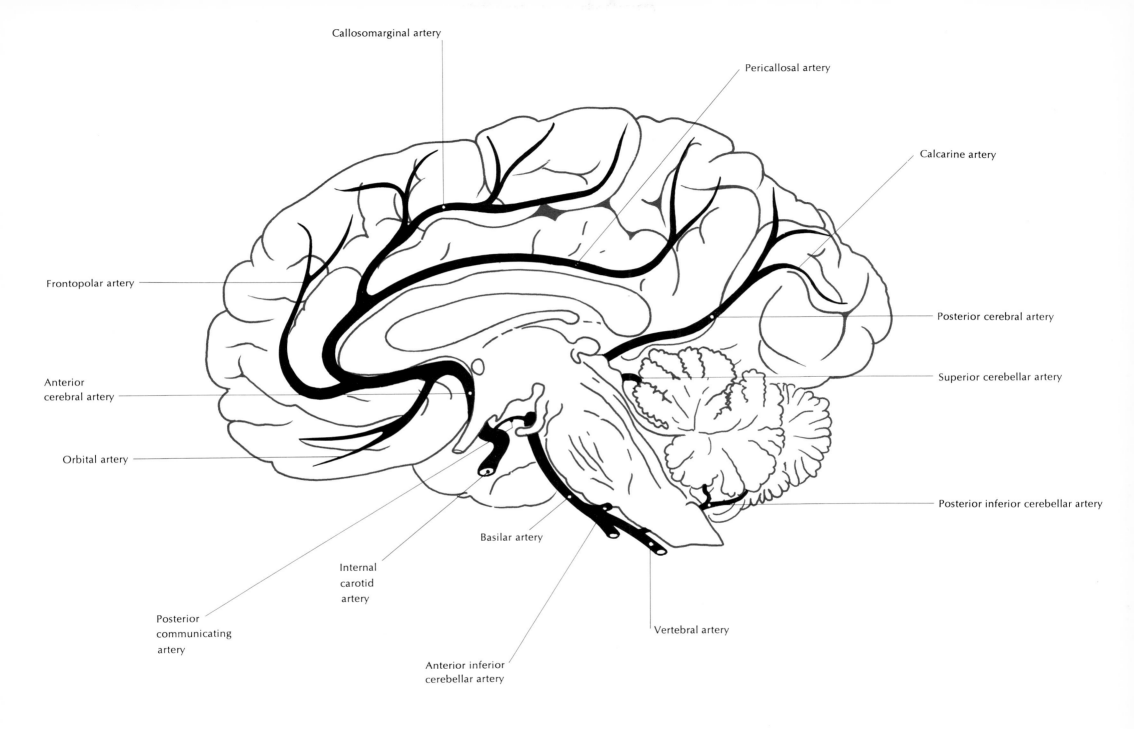

Callosomarginal artery

Pericallosal artery

Calcarine artery

Frontopolar artery

Posterior cerebral artery

Anterior cerebral artery

Superior cerebellar artery

Orbital artery

Posterior inferior cerebellar artery

Basilar artery

Internal carotid artery

Vertebral artery

Posterior communicating artery

Anterior inferior cerebellar artery

Figure 77. Arterial blood supply to the medial surface of the brain

153

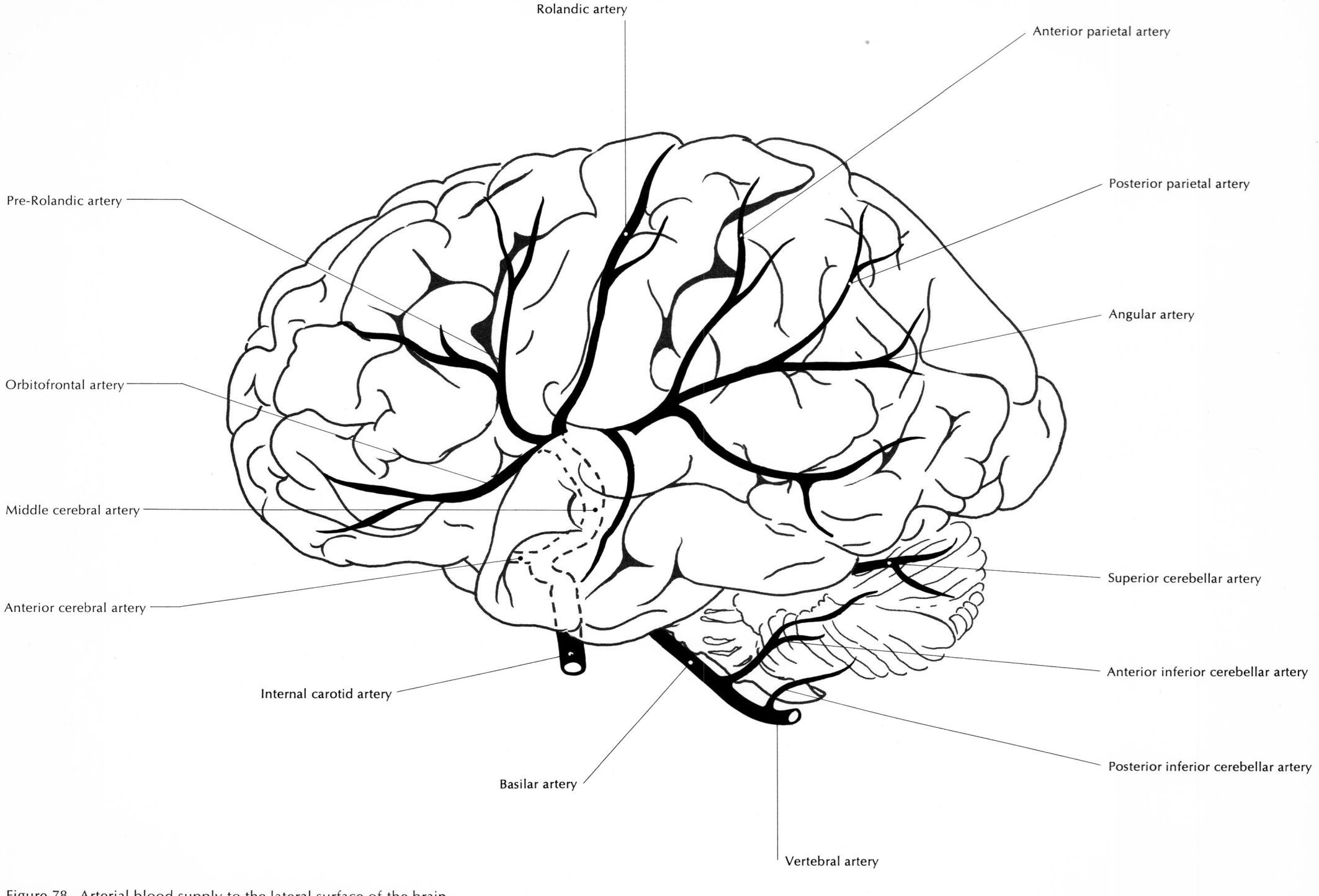

Rolandic artery

Anterior parietal artery

Pre-Rolandic artery

Posterior parietal artery

Orbitofrontal artery

Angular artery

Middle cerebral artery

Anterior cerebral artery

Superior cerebellar artery

Anterior inferior cerebellar artery

Internal carotid artery

Posterior inferior cerebellar artery

Basilar artery

Vertebral artery

Figure 78. Arterial blood supply to the lateral surface of the brain

154

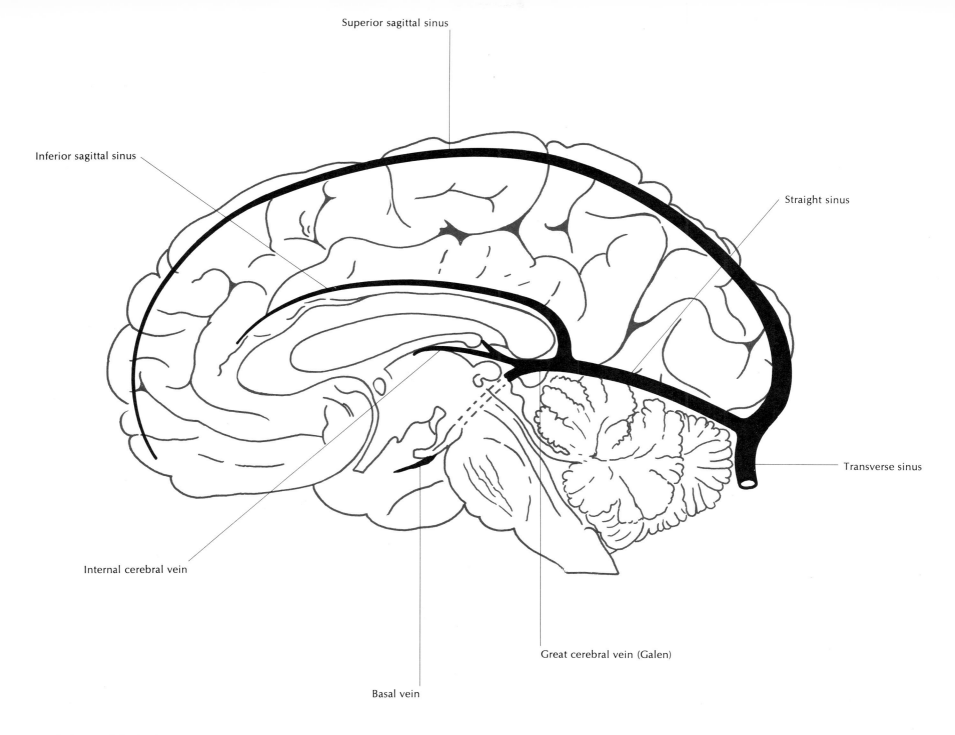

Superior sagittal sinus

Inferior sagittal sinus

Straight sinus

Internal cerebral vein

Transverse sinus

Great cerebral vein (Galen)

Basal vein

Figure 79. Major venous drainage of the brain

155

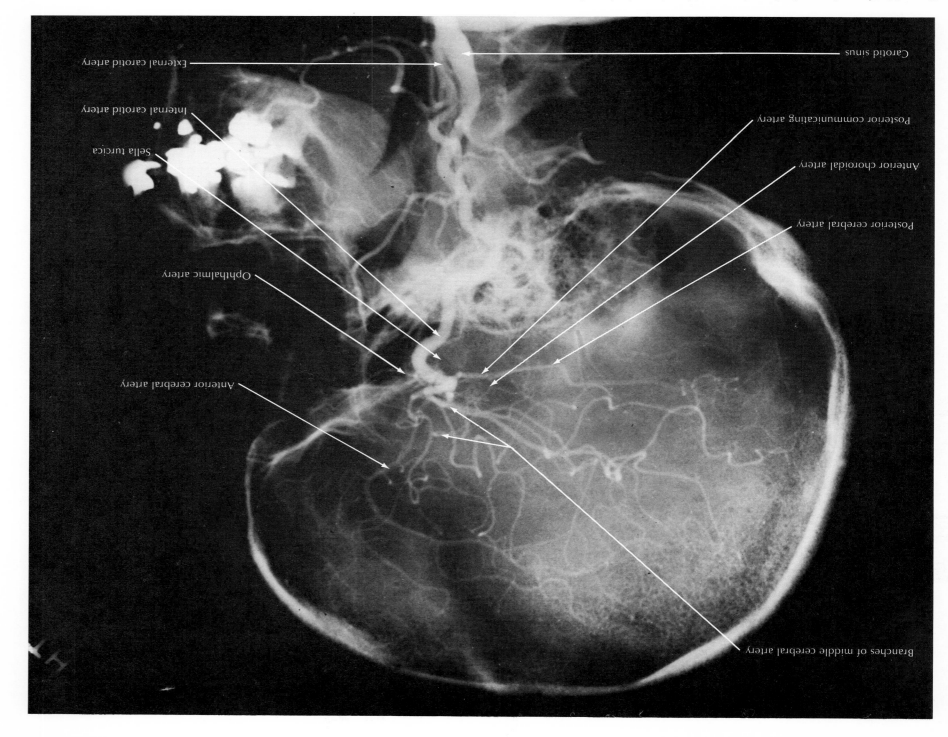

Figure 80. The major cerebral arteries, carotid angiography lateral projection

Carotid sinus

External carotid artery

Internal carotid artery

Sella turcica

Ophthalmic artery

Anterior cerebral artery

Posterior communicating artery

Anterior choroidal artery

Posterior cerebral artery

Branches of middle cerebral artery

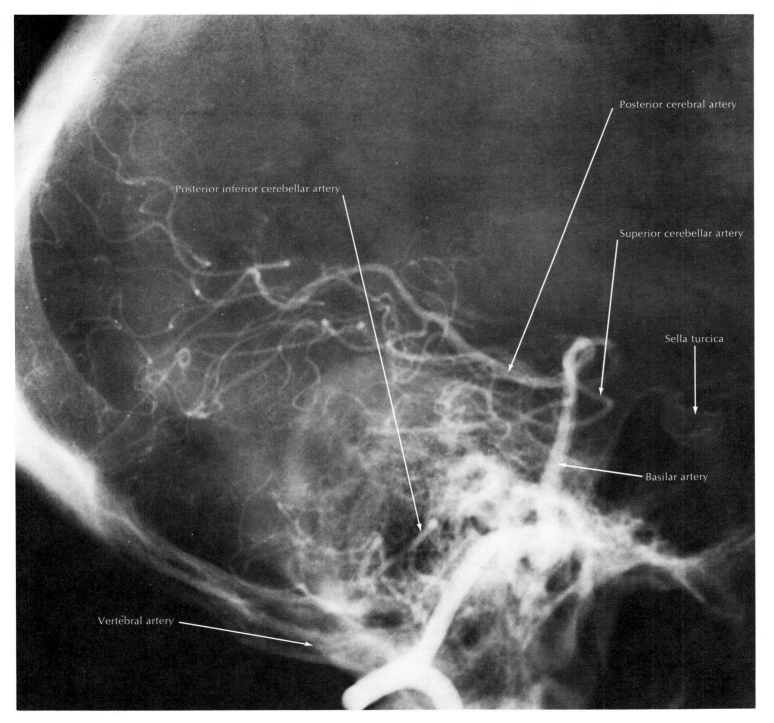

Posterior cerebral artery

Posterior inferior cerebellar artery

Superior cerebellar artery

Sella turcica

Basilar artery

Vertebral artery

Figure 81. The major cerebral arteries, vertebral angiography, lateral projection

157

Figure 82. The major cerebral arteries, carotid angiography, frontal projection

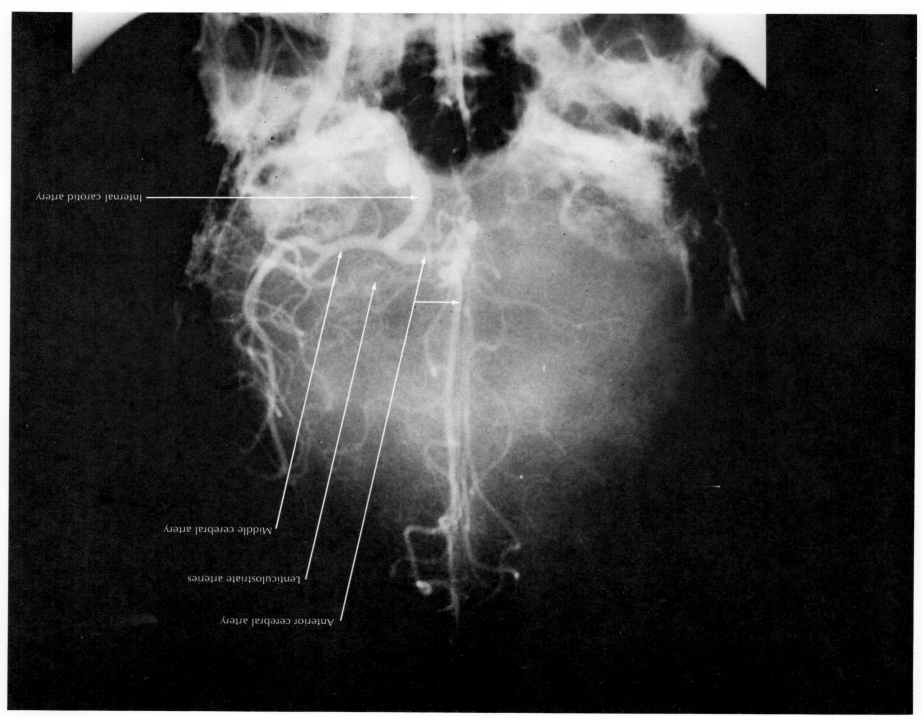

Internal carotid artery

Middle cerebral artery

Lenticulostriate arteries

Anterior cerebral artery

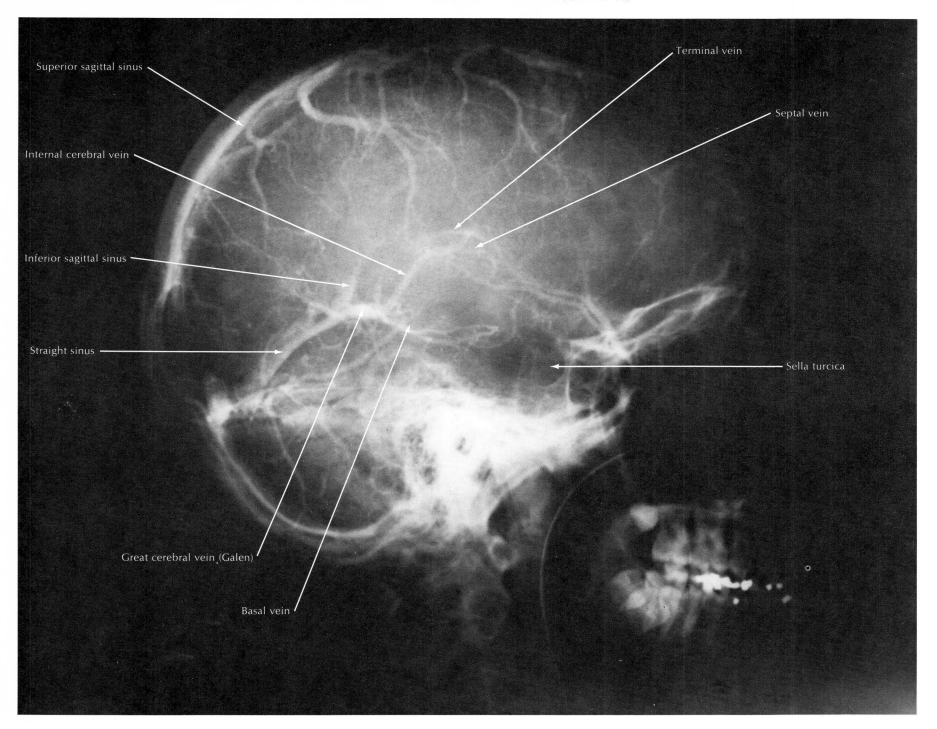

Superior sagittal sinus

Internal cerebral vein

Inferior sagittal sinus

Straight sinus

Great cerebral vein (Galen)

Basal vein

Terminal vein

Septal vein

Sella turcica

Figure 83. The major cerebral veins and dural sinuses, lateral projection

159

Index